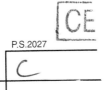

*Jason Tune and Martin Warburton*

**chipmunka**
The mental

Jason Tune

Published by
Chipmunkapublishing
PO Box 6872
Brentwood
Essex CM13 1ZT
United Kingdom

**http://www.chipmunkapublishing.com**

Chipmunkapublishing gratefully acknowledge the support of Arts Council England.

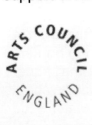

# Foreword: by Dr. Justin Marley

It is a great privilege for me to have been asked by Jason Tune to write this foreword. During my training in psychiatry, I've spent time working with the Rotherham Early Intervention Team while undertaking research. During my time with the team, I've had the great pleasure to have worked with Jason.

On meeting him for the first time I was impressed by his almost limitless energy, boundless enthusiasm for his work and infectious humour. I quickly came to learn that he is well liked by both staff and patients and was surprised to learn that in addition to his work he had found the time to write a very successful book. Now he has written a second book and in this book which he has co-authored with Martin Warburton, Jason combines both courage and generosity. He is courageous in that he reveals very sensitive details about himself, about times which must have been very difficult for him. He is generous in that he does this with a higher purpose in mind - breaking down the barriers that society places in the way of those that suffer with mental illness. Jason tells us candidly about the experience of being shunned within the community because of the label of having a mental illness. He tells us about the different ways in which he was made to feel like an outcast from the community after he was first admitted to a psychiatric ward. Friends that he had known for many years would avoid him; he would be laughed at when applying for work and would have considerable difficulty in developing relationships or even getting served in the pub. Fortunately Jason is extremely resilient and has been able to overcome these many difficulties, to turn this around and help those in the position that he was once in.

There's something more. He doesn't stop but just keeps moving on, learning about himself and helping others in the process in many different ways. In this book he can give hope to others who suffer a mental illness, to show them what is possible even when they are at the lowest point in their lives and when others don't understand what they're going through. For those who have not experienced a mental illness, this book again offers hope, a hope associated with the human spirit which Jason exemplifies in abundance. Martin Warburton has also shown courage in sharing with us his experiences of mental illness and the stigma associated with drug use and he compliments Jason's uplifting story.

## Introduction: by Jason

Since my autobiography "Sex Drugs and Northern Soul" people have asked me about what has happened to me both publicly and professionally. Some of the reviews and the positive feedback from my autobiography have really touched me. One of the questions that I have been asked is how did my mental illness affect me? As I am now working in mental health, I can look back and say that the stigma unfortunately associated with mental illness was for me worse than the episode of the illness.

My aim and hope is to give people an insight into what it feels like to be stigmatised but more significantly, how I challenged perceptions. My work behind the scenes is to promote awareness, to help reduce the ignorance and to go underneath my illness being totally honest about how mental ill health can hold you back. I am not going to say that I will be politically correct or medically correct for that matter. Nor am I going to say that my experiences are comparable to anyone else's experiences.

I am going to illustrate a positive spin from some of the symptoms that often occur during a period of mental ill health. I will also be writing about the support that family and friends gave me over the course of my illness and beyond and I will also mention the support from professionals. I will also be talking about my journey from ill health to recovery and beyond leading to my current job and the roles I now have.

## Acknowledgements

I would like to give a special mention to Alexandra Scott – Mental Health Nutritionist within the Early Intervention Team, who has edited the manuscript. I would also like to thank my colleagues, family and friends who have supported me on this venture.

## Chapter 1: Stigma

Stigma comes in many different forms and my first memory of it was back in 1969 at Kimberworth School Infants in Rotherham aged 4 going on 5 when I had squinty eyes and needed glasses, I was on free school meals and had to queue in a separate queue from the other kids. At this point in my life I obviously had little appreciation of the complexities of the emotions induced by rejection, but for the first time ever I became angry as a result of it and this anger was to be a driving force in my life for some years to come. The big kids, on the same road, who went to the comprehensive school were calling me "Clarence the crossed eyed lion", "Bozz eyed bastard" and other derogative terms associated with my lazy eye. One day I looked over the infant school playground wall into the adjacent comprehensive school yard and promised myself that one day I'm going to be the biggest, toughest guy there and nobody is ever going to bully me again.

As I wrote in my first book that when I went to jumble sales with my grandma, whom I loved dearly and who left me with memories that I would not sacrifice for all the tea in China, I was often seen by older kids who verbally expressed their depreciation of my attire. I preferred to run these evening sorties during winter for the protection of the cover of darkness. However, the love of my gran outweighed the pain of my ignorant persecutors. Although there wasn't much money around at that time in my neck of the woods I was fetched up with a word called "respect" and amongst my peers respect was paramount.

Throughout my primary school days I started going to Sunday school, the Salvation Army and Pentecostal Church, although I wasn't sure about all the things I was being taught in these places I learned enough respect and decent values to feel I had gained something that outweighed the labelling of "Bible basher" and other such derision directed at me by my peers. Nobody likes to be shown up but I recall as a child in the mid seventies being publicly denounced in the swimming baths upon being caught trying to smuggle my verruca into the water. It was always better if one had the chance to share their verrucca with other children as the blame would be diluted and one would not stand alone "a problem shared being a problem halved" and all that.

One memory of my childhood concerns parents not allowing their children to mix because of their backgrounds. A particular painful instance of where I fell foul of this concerned a young lady who had captivated my heart in the last year of primary school yet it could not be due to the non-acceptance of her higher socioeconomic status family who did not approve of the families on my estate. We were disempowered from being able to make our own decisions, the consequences not quite leading to the tragedy of Romeo and Juliet but none-the-less people underestimate the pain that young hearts can feel.

# Stigma: Worse than Psychosis

Into my comprehensive school days, I hadn't realised I had been marked with a reputation that went before me and I feel this reputation did not truly represent who I was. I was the young guy that helped the elderly cross the road, helped his family for love rather than reward, wished to succeed at schoolwork and even did bits of charity work. My misleading reputation and false friends, that clung to me because they enjoyed trouble, brought stigma upon me. I ran into this trap through simply trying to survive.

When I was a child a frequently repeated dictum that I heard was "Sticks and stones may break my bones but words can never harm me". Can I just pause here to ask how many of you readers have never been hurt by words?

In all honesty in the days of my early youth, before I had personally experienced the impact of extreme stigma, in my ignorance, I myself cast the occasional stone. I was one of the gang and a name caller too. Through ignorance I had been involved in name calling directed at individuals affected by poor mental health, although we did not know what made them seem different and be such easy targets at the time. In those days children had little education about psychological bullying and mental health prejudice, which remains inadequately addressed to date, was acceptable to most adults never mind children. Conspicuous figures in my social environment were "Carrier bag Annie" and "Vinegar Liz" who were on the receiving end of our derision Most of the slandering

11

perpetrated by my peers and I was unfounded and indeed "A'tchet Olive" was never actually seen with an axe. The only crime she ever committed was to be sent to various psychiatric institutions during a less unenlightened era. Unfortunately "Tab hunter" did live up to his name but never hurt anyone, I wish the same could be said for our gang.

Many people recall how they themselves were bullies as children until they were bullied which caused them to relate to their own victims, wake up to the pain they were inflicting and for most reasonable people lead them to stop. This phenomenon is not limited to bullying of the physical kind as verbal persecution often results more from ignorance than malice.

In my early life I had no conception of the new kind of stigma that was to be inflicted upon me, disempowering me from such an early age, destroying my self esteem and radically reducing my quality of life for so many years to come. In late December 1980, a month after turning 16, I was admitted to "Rotherham Psychiatric Unit" (as it was known then but now the "Mental Health Unit"). This was a life changing event. The direct impact of my psychiatric health problems was a significant enough blow without being compounded by the devastating aftermath of the stigma. My mental health issues had a serious enough effect on their own, which should not be brushed under the carpet, however, the emphasis of this book is on the stigma generated as a result which I feel has been a much greater problem over the years for both myself and the similarly afflicted.

There I was looking forward to manhood and all the respect that adult life would have to offer and suddenly the future did not look so bright from the inside of a windowless seclusion room. What are my friends at school going to think? One time I avoided them when they came to see me not wanting them to see me in the state I was in and yet I had no reason to believe that my state would improve. I felt that my life was truly over. An eleven year lead-up to the exams and there would be no Jason Tune present, amongst my peers that had not already heard about my great fall questions would be asked. I would also be conspicuous by my absence at leaving celebrations I had once looked forward to whilst I was more immediately preoccupied by the question of when would I get to leave the hospital? I had no control over what was happening to me, and certainly no control over people's perceptions of me or what they said about me to others. The stigma directed at me affected others close to me too, my sister Samantha, who was only 12 years old at the time, being one such casualty. She used to regularly visit me, she was very close to me and years later was to tell me of two tough incidents in which she was forced to stand her ground whilst being taunted about my ill health. One of these taunters was later to have mental health problems herself and become a "revolving door patient" (an unofficial term within the mental health services for someone frequently in and out of hospital).

Unfortunately the losses were great and things had gone from one extreme to another. Many friends had disappeared off the scene. I had always been popular with the girls through my youth club, school and the adult world of Northern Soul music scene, however, if even my female friends were abandoning me how would my romantic pursuits be affected? I can remember going to a pub nearby the hospital, they refused to serve me a glass of coke because they knew I was staying in the hospital and this was at a time when I had little problems being served beer elsewhere. There were certain places I would hear whispers about me relating to the fact that I was a psychiatric patient. This was approximately three decades ago yet even then racial prejudice was frowned upon, in the interim homophobia and prejudice against disabled people have become more frowned upon, however, there is still a long way to go in terms of combating stigma and prejudice surrounding mental health issues with stigmatising words and phrases still being common language.

Once I had got rid of the standard issue hospital foam slippers, dressing gown and pyjamas that never fit (conveniently loose so the Largactil squad could easily whip 'em down to stick a needle in my arse) I was ready to go out on home leave back in my civilian clothing that one is allowed to wear in the free world. Just over 6 months had past before being allowed my first leave and although I felt well enough to be out of the hospital I did not feel well enough to engage within the community. Certainly I had become confident at mastering the environment of the hospital; however, mastery of the outside world, in which I had spent the whole of my life prior to my admission, had somehow become more elusive. This was perhaps made no easier by the timing of my stay being the interlude between childhood and adulthood though I feel a good portion of my difficulties in rejoining wider society at this time could have been avoided had there been rehabilitative input such as there is today.

Thankfully some members of my local community saw me as a person with problems rather than a problem person, unfortunately this was not a universal attitude. A memory I normally try to forget, but which I will now recall as it seems necessary to help the reader gain a useful insight, is that of being called "Frankenstein". This might seem like nothing to most people as practically everyone has been called names they don't like at some point, however, when someone is ill, vulnerable, feels out of control and the issue of their illness is very sensitive the experience is very different. I would have to laugh along with it or things would get worse but all the time it hurt and the amount of extra pain I had to suffer, on top of that directly being caused by my illness, was being decided by and controlled by other people.

After approximately two months at home, in autumn 1981, I set off on what would normally have been a 10 minute walk, which was more like an hour with my Largactil shackles on, down to the canal bank area near the local sewage works. The purpose of this ill fated expedition was to seek work as I had heard a construction firm was recruiting personnel to work on a new sewage system. By this point I had become desperate to be seen as normal and wanted to be one of the lads again. As I walked into the workmen's cabin on their lunch break I was totally unprepared for the barrage of humiliating laugher that was to be directed at me. These sewage workers thought they were clever enough to take the piss but it was no real loss to me, it was a shit job anyway.

At that time, before supermarkets took off the way they have today, local shops were much more of a community focal point. My mother would send me to our local shop on errands. I did not realise it at this time but she was trying to motivate me, prevent me from spending all day in bed and help me recover my confidence. Just as Arabs who almost never meet in the desert might gather at an oasis to trade goods the people of my estate would meet at the shop not just to buy goods but to trade gossip as well. We had been a relatively private family in a tight-knit community in which everyone knew each other's business. Despite our discretion elements of my situation were impossible to conceal and I soon became the focus of much of the shop's tickle tackle information exchange. I developed a painful awareness of this, burned out from the combined effects of my illness and medication, and found it increasingly difficult to brush off. My mother thought I was just becoming lazy, not wanting to go to the shop, but had not grasped the picture. Perhaps I should have told her what I was going through but I did not want to burden my mother with my problems and young men on my estate did not share such things with their mothers, or even anyone else if they could help it, as it did not quite go with the compulsory macho image deemed necessary for survival. Now with my greater maturity I realise how naïve I was in my adolescence and see it as a strength and not a weakness to talk about my feelings and express my emotions in the right circumstances. Many of my female friends even see this as a very positive feature in a man.

The whole business of not being able to discuss my feelings resulted in me becoming an isolated prisoner on my estate with my family and friends being physically all around me but psychologically a million miles away. My situation was such that it was like being in an isolated desert, not a sand or snow desert but a people desert. It is no good people actually being there if one cannot communicate with them in the manner one needs to. Interestingly enough a health care professional I met years later said, whilst referring to those times, "It was like a desert out there" meaning that there was no support in the community for people that had endured such experiences. Once this kind of isolation experience gets a hold it can spiral out of control. Today, in our more enlightened but still imperfect times, there is help out there and I implore people to make immediate use of these services at the first sign of danger of isolation getting a hold. There are professionals out there that one can discuss issues with that one may be reluctant to speak of in everyday social circles.

However, back in the early 1980's things were very different. The stigma I had to bear was disabling me in that I was reluctant and embarrassed to be seen in my social environment and yet, as any human does, I still needed social contact. My confidence was reduced to the point that I was rarely able to seek out the people who had been my friends and they almost never made the effort to seek out my company. Occasionally I would see an old associate who used to be eager to be seen with me at the youth club, or wherever else, when I was top dog on the estate and they would cross the road so as to not have to walk past me. It was unclear whether they would be embarrassed to be seen with me or if they were afraid of the mentally ill monster. I had been in the army cadets with many local lads and we had talked about being blood brothers and so forth the way that teenagers do. Where were these mates now? Would I have really wanted to have trusted these lads with my life in the trenches? I'm alright Jack and all that. Some of these guys had been working on my estate at this time, carrying out renovations, and had even been on my street but not one of them ever called by to ask how I was. I had seen various other lads who had been friends waiting at the bus stop on my road, often with their girlfriends, and they did not even look into my house. To me it seemed everyone else who was moving on with their lives, had left me behind and I was outside this normality.

## Stigma: Worse than Psychosis

Prior to my illness my mother's phone never stopped ringing with people eager to make social arrangements and after the onset of my illness the phone would still ring, my heart beat accelerating with anticipation and hope, but the call would never be for me. A small number of friends had visited me in hospital, including a particularly loyal friend called Julie, but generally speaking I had become a social leper from the moment of my admission and nothing had changed upon my discharge. In truth I had done some of the avoiding myself, through feelings of shame and low self esteem, though all the while yearning for the company of people that perhaps had never really been my friends. As for their part some may have not known how to relate to me feeling awkward or even afraid but I think most simply felt, at best, they had more to gain investing their time in other people and, at worst, that being associated with me was a liability.

This period, simply the interlude between my first hospital stay and the relapse leading to my second, was to be the last time that I lived on the estate upon which I grew up. I moved on having invested the best part of 16 years of my social life into those few streets and left with no returns.

In stark contrast to my experiences in friendships, my relatives were extremely supportive and caring. What they lacked in experience of dealing with mental illness they naturally made up for with love. Often I did not feel like I deserved this love as I believed I had brought shame upon our family and let everyone down. I felt I could give nothing of any value in return. I felt as though I was a burden to them and could see no positives to my illness or its knock-on effects. In those days the words "recovery" or "positive" were almost never used in the mental health services and one did not have contact with the kind of staff whose role it is to use them today. My extreme difficulties and my subjective feelings of failure to survive, even on my home ground, led to a voluntary admission back to hospital in the winter of 1981, just before Christmas and only a few months after I had been discharged. This time I was in such a state I did not need any help from the authorities to gain entry to what was to become my favoured hotel whilst wishing to take a break in the Don Valley Riviera.

There was some relief in admitting I could not cope in the community, as it meant I no longer had to endure the agony of trying and the fear of failure meant nothing once I had failed. It was one year on from the point at which I had seriously wanted to be a soldier and I was a casualty without ever having had chance to join the ranks.

## Chapter 2: Medications

Psychotropic medications are far from perfect today but some can work for some people usually with the cost of side effects. In the early eighties most of the medications were different, indeed some would work to lessen the symptoms they were intended to treat in patients lucky enough to respond, but whether they were effective at treating the symptoms they were targeted at or not enduring the side effects was often a horrific ordeal. The Jason Tune that had been the youth club Jack-the-lad and centre of attention never short of a girl on his arm had now somehow metamorphosed into a several stone overweight, unshaven being with saliva drooling down its chin and little ability to bend its limbs and body, only able to walk like a zombie. Thank God I'm back to my usual handsome self now. Strangely enough I appeared to be developing a phobia of mirrors during this period.

Much of this time the drug of choice, not my choice but the choice of the psychiatrists, was Largactil. This was more formally known as "Chlorpromazine" which is well renowned for causing almost paralytic muscle stiffening and its effects on one's gait. Throughout much of the Western world, due to this effect upon a person's gait, a person experiencing this common side effect of this drug is formally referred to as doing the "Chlorpromazine waltz", however, in the slightly less formal locality of Rotherham it is generally known as the "Largactil shuffle". On reflection I wonder whether this drug does incur any therapeutic benefits at all, or whether it is simply given to patients in psychiatric units to make them easier to spot and catch should they ever get out. I won't insult the reader's intelligence here by going into details about how the effects of such a drug impact upon stigma as it is easy to understand how such afflicted individuals appear. It is, however, worth drawing attention to the point that any such individual has no real possibility of maintaining any self esteem and their self-image would be likely to be a constant source of pain. Would you want to date such a person? Well that might not actually matter to them as much as you thought as this drug often destroys its takers libido (if they are lucky as all too often it can render a man impotent whilst they still have their libido in tact). I am afraid I know less about its effects on women as I have been too polite to ask.

Largactil must have had some benefits otherwise the psychiatrists would not have prescribed it. Unfortunately, as patients were usually too embarrassed to mention sexual dysfunction side effects or at least the full extent and discomfort of these effects, when it came to the psychiatrists weighing up the benefits verses deficits of prescribing such a drug the equation was prone to being improperly balanced. Largactil is far less commonly used today largely being replaced by drugs with a better ratio of pros to cons. Thankfully now, with the times being a little more enlightened, more having been learned about side effects and perhaps a better atmosphere on the wards due to a more client centred approach, it is a little easier for most patients to discuss sexual dysfunction.

The delights of Largactil did not end there and the list of physical side effects was bad enough without the ones that exacerbated the stigma. Largactil and some other drugs make people extremely light sensitive and prone to sunburn. In the summers of the early Eighties I could not go outside without being smeared in sun cream even on days when no one else could get burned even if they tried. This made me even more conspicuous. Such phenomena, that visibly mark people, give patients who are often suffering from paranoia something genuine to worry about.

At any one time in the hospital many if not most people with psychosis were given this drug. It was as though we were all treading grapes as we hobbled along. Whatever the logic behind this was it really appeared to be a one size fits all medication solution. A lot of psychiatrists have had their favourite medications that they liked to prescribe widely as they believed they were the most effective. With today's more client centred approach the individual's pharmacological response to medication seems to be given greater attention and with, perhaps, a wider range of psychotropic drugs being available the psychiatrist has more options.

"God do these people know what they're doing?" "Do they know how much pain they are causing me?" I thought as a team of burley, asylum trained, psychiatric nurses, injected a generous helping of Largactil into my rear and hurled me into a pharmaceutical dungeon. Such people did not know the suffering induced by the side effects, either those deemed "normal" or those experienced by a susceptible individual that had extra dimensions to their hell, but they pretty much did know that the rest of their shift would be easier. Adolescence is ordinarily a time of protesting about this, that and the other for young people with the most mundane of lives. A person with 20:20 vision might well have trouble finding a needle in a haystack but place an adolescent in Utopia and they will find something to protest about. Well I wasn't quite in Utopia, my accommodation wasn't quite the Ritz and, without wishing to criticise all the staff, for some part the service was appalling. I could cope with dinner not being served on a silver platter but the way they served my night-cap in a syringe was somehow unpalatable, not to mention that this night-cap was sometimes served during the day and was always involuntary room service.

The physical pain and people exercising power over me were not the only things I was protesting against, I was also aware that these people were inflicting effects upon me that marked me, made me vulnerable to ridicule, eliminated any chance of getting a girlfriend and annihilated my self esteem. I would be thrown into a darkened room but there would be no need to lock the door behind me as my chemical prison would be enough. This was easier than talking to me. To me it simply seemed like a great injustice as I was being punished for being ill rather than for any wrongdoing. The fact that I was in a hospital, where people are supposed to be cared for, added dimensions of bewilderment and distrust of society to my ordeal. There were some decent nurses on the ward but still today I think it is unlikely that the actions of the people forcing my chemical straightjacket on me were motivated by aims of rehabilitation. My protests were mostly verbal and I was not particularly polite, but sometimes physical too as I tried to stop them doing whatever it was they were trying to do with me at the time. After a certain point the stress induced by the sight of the "Largactil squad", as they were known in the hospital at the time, would cause me the kind of agitation that I was supposed to be given the drug for.

Soon I was approaching the Largactil squad and asking for the drug, I seemed to have become addicted to having it at a certain time and my requests also gave me some control over the situation and took power out of their hands. Eventually, through a hap-hazard route, my protesting paid off. The one time I actually fought the Largactil squad I was sent for a long stay in seclusion and was put under a different psychiatrist who tried me with a different drug. Bingo, she hit the target perfectly, for the first time ever I realised that psychiatric medications can be a great help, one just needs the right drug, and I was never subjected to the Largactil needle or seclusion ever again.

## Chapter 3: "You shouldn't be in a place like this at your age!"

Am I one of these people? I thought as I looked around me at the other mentally ill people I was sharing this rehabilitation ward with. It was early 1984 and I had been admitted to a rehabilitative psychiatric ward that was different from the acute wards that I had previously experienced. Here resided many long-term mentally ill people, the so-called "revolving door patients", and there was no one in my age group to relate to with the rest of the clientele all being older adults.

There were lots of scary looking people all around, pacing up and down, sat around tables and staring at this, that, the other and into space (best not to stare back). The population of this new environment were clad in bizarre attire often including half-mast trousers or pyjamas and other such trademarks that marked them as belonging to this new world. I felt I had lost my way and wandered into an unfamiliar land tainted by a sinister enchantment. Though I had never suffered a lack of imagination my nightmares had previously always failed to conjure up such a horror setting as was now my living environment.

The ward was much cleaner than the language used in it with the powerful aroma of disinfectant hanging in the air a permanent feature, competing only with the cigarette smoke smog in the lounge. Through this smoky mist one could see the figures of often bedraggled, weather-beaten folk that looked somehow surreal. At least that's how it appeared through young, astounded eyes. The asylums had recently closed, there were no secure units in the nearby area and so their old occupants had found themselves here and were quite possibly marvelling as much at my strangeness as I theirs. The general situation was such that there was ultimately a very diverse range of patients upon the ward with this diversity included dimensions such as diagnosis and time spent in the system. The inevitability of this was that extremely vulnerable people had to rub shoulders with highly exploitative survivors, who had been in the system a long time, and the highly anxious with the highly aggressive.

Juveniles would not be allowed in such an environment today but this juvenile had to find a way to get through it. It would be a major task considering the old hands at work here, who often had known each other a long time, with ancient alliances formed and impenetrable cliques established.

Due to previous incidents on the acute wards, whereby I had to evade being homosexually assaulted and another whereby a paedophile began telling me the intricacies of his favourite activities, I had concluded that I did not wish to share a dorm with anyone and my high anxiety levels constantly reminded me of this point. It came as a considerable relief when I was give my own room almost straight away, maybe everyone else was too scared to share with me eh?

Even by this time, only 3 to 4 years after being in the system, in addition to my psychiatric illness, I had begun to develop the disease of institutionalisation. This was obviously a highly contagious affliction, as almost all my neighbours on the ward were affected. Though they had all seemed so strange and outlandish to me, I was similarly marked by so many of the trademark clichés from the clothing to weight gain, not to mention the behavioural and psychological traits. Part of my rehabilitation involved social inclusion. This was in some ways a good idea and certainly well intended, but also had its drawbacks. My attempts to avoid people knowing I was going to and from the hospital involved much effort and were often very creative, but this was an uphill struggle as I was more marked than a sitting duck with a target tattooed on its arse. I would avoid catching the bus in the hospital grounds or the one that said "Hospital" in the bus station. It involved an awful lot of effort and if I was lucky I could pass myself off as just a fat guy with no dress sense.

Many of the folk inhabiting this strange new land of the long-stay rehabilitation wards had lived in the old asylums for a considerable time. They were veterans of many a squabble with the more able amongst them being impeccable negotiators, adept at intimidation, and had survival down to a fine art. To be a babe in these woods would be very unfortunate indeed; I was not going to be a babe.

Many of the patients had resided in the same asylum before being transferred to the Rotherham psychiatric unit. These people had had a long time to form bonds, made all the stronger for the shared hardships they had endured together and they had learned who the strong and useful allies were. At the time of my arrival on these wards there was a kind of established mob running the show. Underground activities included bookkeeping for the horses, gambling over pool, cards and table tennis, cigarette baroning and whatever else would basically yield a profit. Our bookkeeper saved us from having to make the precarious journey to the bookies in town along the route of which one could be molested by bigots and exposed to the ravages of stigma. Attempts were made to carry out the many illicit transactions discreetly and in all the time I was on the wards I don't recall anyone ever being caught. All punters had to be vetted before being allowed to partake in such business ventures, "grasses strictly not allowed" and whether this strict security worked or whether the nursing staff simply had bigger fish to fry I leave you, the reader, to decide.

Unbeknown to me gambling was not restricted to events on the TV and I wandered up to a pool match boisterously and asked if I could take the winner on. This was a best of three matches with ten whole cigarettes at stake and tensions were high. In my early naïvety I had lit a powder keg, or at least that could be one way of describing the experience of being suddenly being hit with a pool cue and a moment later another, from one of the opposing player. It turned out that these two individuals were nicknamed "the dangerous brothers" and I never wasted too much time trying to puzzle out why. Perhaps surviving the incident alone would have been a feat beyond the capabilities of many, but when I came out on top it was a great achievement which automatically gave me the position of ward "cigarette baron". A packet of twenty cigarettes in those days cost about a pound, each cigarette would be sold for ten pence and being the head entrepreneur in this field guaranteed my nicotine supply and solvency throughout the rest of my stay. The days of the staff rationing my cigarettes, keeping them for me allowing me one per hour as they did on the acute wards, were a fading memory.

The tobacco empire was mine but it was not the only principality. For example the world of playing cards belonged to another. He was not a military dictator by any means whatsoever but was a shrewd bounder who could sense any card-related opportunity with uncanny ESP-like abilities and bought into the general rule of the place that minor exploitation was simply a means of surviving boredom and poverty. The occupational therapy room, adjacent to the ward, served as both the pool room and the table tennis room. Table tennis games were normally played for a twenty pence stake with the winner staying on; however, the play was not always fair. The king that was holding court over the table tennis racket was known as "Zippy". Whereas the tactics of most players centred on how they would hit the ball, it was not necessarily only the ball that Zippy was thinking of hitting. He wanted you to know that! He was most displeased when I was taking the lead in the first game I ever played with him and resorted to threats that basically involved a weapon and unpleasant death. This led to a fight in which, thankfully, no weapon was actually used and I emerged the victor. After this we sort of became pals and played many a less eventful game of table tennis. It would be nice to say that I won them all but unfortunately that was definitely not the case.

One of my favourite sporting activities, that also provided a temporary escape from the ward, was swimming. We used to go to the local leisure centre and the lady who usually took us was stunningly beautiful, caring, sensitive and respectful towards people with mental illness which were all well appreciated traits. At some point most men find themselves harbouring affections for some nurse or nurse-like figure that they encounter by whatever unfortunate circumstances, as vulnerable people are susceptible to emotional triggers and may be prone to great positive regard towards someone meeting their needs, especially if that person is a beautiful young woman. Well this young lady stands out as possibly the nurse-like figure that I most appreciated. When going swimming with a group I did feel the sting of the stigma as it was so apparent to any viewer that we were not typical members of the public. However, sometimes there would be just me and her going, no one would suspect anything or particularly notice me and everything would be right in the world, at least until our return to the ward. I was not obsessed with this woman but the peace and feeling of wellbeing I had when there was only the two of us present felt such a stark contrast to life in the hospital.

There was also a gym in the hospital, that was available to us twice each week and using this was an important part of my journey to recovery, rebuilding my self esteem and helping me to resist the effects of the omnipresent stigma. I can't begin to recommend enough a good workout in the gym for stress relief and its therapeutic powers helped me workout many of my issues and get me through this difficult period. Soon I was involved in a "Back to work" group, which basically was intended to prepare us for re-entering the world of work. It involved several projects; all supervised by a member of mental health service staff, including preparations for psychiatric patients leaving the hospital to live in their own homes out in the community, such as decorating and moving furniture.

We also had a "Greenhouse project", growing fresh vegetables and a "Carwash project" amongst others. The greenhouse was good for encouraging us to consume more fresh vegetables and it was certainly known then how good they were for physical health, however, since then there has been an increasing momentum of evidence emerging about their benefits for mental health too, including psychosis. My current work with the Early Intervention Team focuses on young people experiencing psychosis. Our multidisciplinary team has nutritionists on board as the benefits of good nutrition in mental health are beginning to be realised and adequate amounts of certain nutrients, have been found to reduce the severity of the psychotic episode. Omega 3 fatty acids, found in oily fish, and some vitamins and minerals have been proven to be beneficial to brain health, function and wellbeing; whilst saturated fat, sugar and caffeine have a negative impact on mood and mental health. It is also of paramount importance that psychiatric patients have the correct advice to help minimise weight gain, or even loss, resulting from side effects of medication not just from a physical health or self image point of view but to help them escape being marked, looking abnormal in a branded kind of way and becoming obvious targets for stigma.

These were the days before channel 4 not to mention all day TV. Whilst sat in the lounge being surrounded by zombie like, under stimulated, vacated minds focused on the test card on the box in the corner of the room (ok I wasn't just surrounded by 'em I was one o' the buggers.....anyhow...) I had an instance of almost, but not quite, divine inspiration. I thought what about our back-to-work group having a carwash project and surely it will be a bit more interesting than spending so much time in this brain atrophying state. The more facets the back-to-work group could explore the more time we could be occupied as the way things had been if a person without psychiatric issues was admitted to the ward it wouldn't be long until they had them (could this explain the personalities of the staff? But most of them were very sweet with their eccentricities).

The profits from the carwash partly went back into the project; some went into activities for us such a camping trip we went on and the remainder went to us as reward money. This project was very productive not only in terms of the funding it yielded, but also in terms of the effects of providing stimulation, facilitating higher self esteem and possibly even preparing people for a possible re-entry back to working life.

Unfortunately whilst we were washing the cars people knew that we were psychiatric patients and we were very visible. I recall one time when I hid in the shed to avoid being seen by someone off the estate I had grown up on. It was not only for my sake that I wished to avoid being seen but I was also trying to protect my family from being further stigmatised. Since these times my two eldest sisters have told me that people did not speak to them much about me and they were not particularly aware of a stigma being attached to our family. However, I had wished to take no chances of my family getting any more trouble than could be helped and my actions may have minimised the danger and spared them overt problems. Although my sisters were unaware of any significant stigma they still would not have known what was being said about our family when they were not present.

It might be nice to tell about how all the poor, nice psychiatric patients, who were always good, were persecuted by all the nasty, ignorant, bigoted, prejudiced members of the public, who were always bad and never had a mental illness; it would be very simple too. However, it very much would not be how things were. The most obvious thing to state, and perhaps something any reader would be already aware of, is that certainly not all members of the public, even then, were prejudiced against people with mental health problems. A slightly less obvious point is that people often don't realise how prejudiced and discriminatory psychiatric patients can be against other psychiatric patients who are in some way different. Even my co-author tells me that sometimes in certain situations, when taken by surprise, shocked, frustrated, angry, upset finds himself bellowing out a barrage of mental illness related discriminatory, abusive terms simply because alternative ways of expressing himself either don't spring to mind quickly enough or would be deemed weird.

For example if one was sitting having a quiet drink in a pub and someone was attacked without apparent warning it is very likely that within the next second or two when describing the assailant people will use adjectives like "nutter" and "sick", instead of saying this person was very violent or bad. Such a response is automatic in our culture, people are conditioned to respond in this way, as though all extreme negative behaviours are to be associated with mental illness, as though no other explanation were possible and this is how mentally ill people behave. People could not express themselves using more accurate terms without having more time to think about it, as they are so unused to it, and even if someone was able to their audience would be so taken aback by their unusual response, that they might think that they were a "nutter", as their word choice would seem outlandish to the masses.

The crowd on any such ward very rarely behaves like one big happy family of individuals within a persecuted minority group, all supporting each other against the pressures of the outsiders persecuting them. In fact it is ordinarily the case that the patients are as far from identifying with all the other patients as Sheffield United Football fans are from liking Sheffield Wednesday fans. Several dimensions of division and discrimination are commonplace, including the able not wanting to be associated with the less able, the non-violent not wanting to be associated with the violent and vice versa, the clean distancing themselves from the dishevelled, the substance users and non-substance users each looking down on the other and the all the other divisions may be present that exist in wider society. It might not seem unreasonable that someone who is moderately depressed or has recently buckled under the stresses of life may not wish to be closely associated with someone spending all day rocking backwards and forwards in a chair, drooling saliva down their chin and making incoherent utterances, however, some folk can be downright insensitive or even cruel about it. Such phenomena are found in most psychiatric wards and the one I was on failed to be an exception. A small number of people on the ward were unfortunate enough to have mild learning disabilities in addition to their mental health issues, and this made them particularly vulnerable to abuse. Insults hurled at these people included "nutcase", nutter, "headbanger", "schizo" and "psycho" all of which anyone with a mental illness could be called out in the community.

There were some characters around however that displayed no fear of stigma or prejudice. I remember one middle-aged lady exclaiming "I have been a prostitute, I have been destitute and now I'm in a f***ing institute!" Unfortunately many amongst the rest of us were far more sensitive. The lady in question was a character I will never forget and her claims to be a "psychic" not a "psychiatric" rather intrigued me. She soon attracted an audience with her electric, larger-than-life presence and gathered in the punters for a variety of money making schemes from palm reading to tarot card reading; I suspect she had the odd scheme going relating to her previous trade but I never needed to be a customer as the food wasn't the only treat I was getting for free in there (from women nearer my age of course).

During the period from my first stay on the long-term wards to my last stay, which included sizable intervals out in the community, I had many flings with other psychiatric patients but had little success with non-mentally ill women. It was nice to have the success I did have and I very much appreciated what the psychiatric patients had to offer but it remained a source of frustration that non-mentally ill women were rarely interested. Some of the women I was involved with were nice enough but when both parties have a significant mental illness things can be complicated. There is often the issue of one or both of you needing someone to cling to and behaving in a manner you would otherwise not. Had I met some of these women after either of us or both of us had recovered, things could have been radically different. There I was left with the issues I had, having realised that attempts at relationships with other patients were not working and with my awareness of my inability to attract other women which led to a significant feeling of disempowerment and hopelessness. The effects the stigma had destroyed my confidence, thus impairing my ability to charm women, which was all too often purely academic as I couldn't even muster the courage to talk to them in the first place.

A particularly clear memory of experiencing the sting of stigma and people's ignorance was that of a day when a group of us were taken to the local polling station to cast our votes and have our say in how things should be done. During our brief time at the polling station, other voters discussed us in an insulting way whilst we were within hearing distance. They must have either thought we were too stupid to tell what they were saying or that what we thought simply did not matter. The terms they used were incredibly derogatory and discriminatory but in the early to mid-Eighties ideas about political correctness were far less developed and people could use such terms and not only be considered to still be good people, but would often be considered to be speaking the views of the majority. A general idea that came across seemed to be that we should not be voting and influencing what was going on in their country, in fact some of them actually said we should not be voting, phrasing it in a most unpleasant and well audible way.

One thing I did very much have in common with many of the other patients was my desire to leave the ward, in a manner that would not result in the police bringing me back, but in a legitimate way. The great master plan I concocted involved me getting myself a Mohican hairstyle in order to get kicked off the ward. Well ok the observant reader may see that this plan might not quite be failsafe but I had the memory of it having caused several of my friends to get kicked out of school....mmm...well maybe it wasn't quite the same thing. I may as well have been trying to get kicked out of Parkhurst prison for refusing to take a library book back, the logic was similar, but in my desperate state I couldn't quite see that at the time. This was kind of my way of registering a protest, far more civilised than smearing excrement on the walls or anything like that and less unpleasant to be involved in, but I am a still a little unsure as to how much impact I actually made.

Despite being unhappy at my stay at this residence, my protest was quite restrained possibly as, since the Largactil squad had left my backside alone for some time by this point, I was a good deal less angry than I had been and even had good relationships with quite a number of the staff. This contrast in how I expressed my displeasure bears testimony to how much my earlier treatment had disturbed me, and been counter-productive by serving to make me angrier. It was such a shock to a sixteen-year-old that had seen little of the world outside school. Healthcare professionals I have met over recent years have expressed the opinion that the treatment I received was barbaric. Thankfully regulations governing such practices today are far stricter.

# Chapter 4: Back in the community

The time came for me to be discharged from the ward and I was sent to live in a hostel near Rotherham town centre. I meant no disrespect to the other clientele but many of them had learning disabilities and though I had some ability to empathise with their plight, I did not wish to be seen as the same or begin to see myself as one of them, at a time when I was trying to re-integrate into the community and raise my self esteem. On reflection, I can now see how my own views have and can be influenced by the stigmas.

At least I was able to go for a drink with my father, the food was good and there were other freedoms but I generally felt alien to the place and avoided activities. There was one time I was briefly romantically involved with a girl from the community but there was no way I could let her know where I lived. My days of cigarette baroning had been left behind on the ward but my reputation had followed me. Due to reward money I was earning on the carwash, I had acquired a large number of cigarettes and there were suspicions I had not done this by legitimate means. This led to my room being searched thoroughly giving me a sense of powerlessness as my privacy was being blatantly invaded right in front of me, with no regard for my thoughts or feelings. Despite this vulgar intrusion, the staff there were generally quite good and one of the few saving graces of the place.

In the mental health services at that time the "token economy system" was still in place, although not as big a feature as it had been in the Sixties and Seventies and rewards would often be given for chores. As I felt so bad about the place I did not want to join in with chores and activities thus reducing my opportunities to earn these rewards in the actual hostel. The rewards I earned were from doing the carwash which was unconnected to the hostel and I managed to stay involved with the carwash as I was still a day patient of the hospital. The hostel afforded me privileges in the form of freedoms. For example I was able to go to the gym with my father and get out into the community to engage in some activities that I had not had the opportunity to do whilst on the ward. On the whole it seemed that life was a little better than on the ward because of the improved chances of engaging within the community, however, being in the hostel itself and the stigma associated with living there was terrible.

Soon I was given a place to live semi-independently which was basically a lodge in the hospital grounds. Although in the hospital grounds, as opposed to being near the town centre as the hostel was, it afforded me greater freedom, as the mental health service staff did not actually work there, but merely checked up on us from time to time and were within reach if we needed them. It was a pleasant change after my three years of ward life and gave me a taste of freedom again. Even little things like having my own letters arriving through a letterbox made a difference. Having my own kitchen and doing my own shopping represented a radical change for the better as I could choose what and when I wanted to eat. I had a television and a three piece suite, things which most people take for granted, but they were new to me, they were mine and they were great. I suppose it's the old story of not appreciating things until you lose them; well I had got them back!

I shared this abode with my housemate, who had been the ward bookkeeper and a few of the patients on the ward would often drop in to place a bet. This guy had been on a Home Office section whilst on the ward and he too was enjoying the novelty of freedom. This Home Office section involved him having to have a compulsory stay on the ward, being brought back by the police should he abscond, and it was a lengthy stay. Similar Home Office sections are decided by the courts. Some Mental Health Act sections involve compulsory stays, and 'Home Office Orders' in particular can be extremely lengthy. Many of the patients I knew who were on sections experienced an acceptable enough degree of recovery to be re-integrated into the community. This guy I shared the lodge and many on other sections were also people that I really enjoyed meeting. However, many people's view of people detained under the Mental Health Act is tainted. There is a great stigma attached to being compulsorily admitted under the Mental Health Act; such that even amongst psychiatric inpatients themselves the voluntary patients often regard themselves as superior, whether they think they are saner or less deviant, than the involuntary patients.

Just as in the media one rarely hears about the operations that go right, people rarely hear about the people with serious mental health problems, many of whom are sectioned at some point, who recover. Just as we hear about the small minority of physical health related operations that go wrong, if someone with a serious mental health problem commits a serious offence, the media particularly focusing on acts of violence, it makes the headlines and colours the public's view of people with such issues. Over recent years there has been a lot of publicity given to any killings whereby the killer had schizophrenia and such newspaper articles often seem to infer that the killer should not have been free to commit the crime in the first place, concomitantly inferring to an often naïve public that all schizophrenic individuals are potential killers. Well indeed all people with schizophrenia are potential killers, as are all human beings including the most mentally healthy amongst us, but when a mentally healthy person kills the tendency is that the media pay little or no attention to the fact that the killer is mentally healthy and do not promote panic that all mentally healthy people are likely to be killers. Needless to mention they do not infer that all mentally healthy people should not be free in the first place to have a chance to kill. It is already a known fact that schizophrenic people are more likely to become the victims of crime than to be the perpetrators. People with schizophrenia make up 1% of the British population, so it would be interesting to know if they really are responsible for more than 1% of unlawful killings. Thankfully I do not have schizophrenia and never became that chronically unwell, it being a terrible affliction often described as "the cancer of the psychiatric world", but I have had a taste of the stigma they have to live with and believe me on top of the suffering they already have to endure they just don't need it.

These people enduring schizophrenia are often amongst the most persecuted individuals on any psychiatric ward, largely due to a combination of their vulnerability and the scaremongering induced reputation associated with their illness. If someone has been given a Mental Health Act section they are frequently assumed to have more serious issues, be less trustworthy and also are prone to becoming the persecuted amongst the persecuted. Some folk really believe that it is the end of someone once they have been sectioned, as these forlorn wretches have deteriorated beyond the point of a reasonable hope of recovery. Many also believe voluntary stay patients should not have to share the same wards with such people, whether because they think they are excessively dangerous, deviant or disgusting to be around and often voluntary stay patients themselves hold this view. However, sectioned patients are a very heterogeneous group, it is usually inappropriate to blame them for their misfortune and believe me they can also be amongst the most vulnerable people on the ward. Patients on sections are often not doomed at all; the section can benefit them and it often represents a turning point in their lives in which they receive the treatment they need. Such people, if they receive appropriate treatment, often get through the immediate crisis and become empowered to exact further positive change, leading to a significant degree of recovery and massively increasing their degree of control over the rest of their lives, and in turn escaping the firm clutches of the stigma into the bargain. As more has been learned over time, this process has improved particularly over the last three decades or so but some great successes were seen back in the 1980's at the time I observed it all first hand. Unfortunately no matter how well a sectioned patient or any other psychiatric patient for that matter recovers there will always be people that remember their darkest times and this keeps the memory of their illness alive through the medium of gossip; one never entirely escapes the stigma.

Just when you think it's safe to go back into the community..... .Whilst out and about in the community something would always catch up with me, for example not being allowed into a pub because the manager knew of my mental health history, or running into people who knew intricate embarrassing details about me at inopportune moments, such as when with a girlfriend. Other guys have even spoken about my mental illness behind my back to deliberately prevent me from getting together with women I have really liked. Whilst living in the lodge I felt less stigmatised than I had felt on the ward; however staff wearing their badges with key chains hanging out of their pockets would come and check up on us regularly. They were very conspicuous and gave the game away immediately that we were not just any members of the community. Our location was very visible being next to the main entrance of the hospital and on a busy road and so many people would have worked out what the house was being used for and seen us coming and going.

I was supposedly back in the community to enable me to re-integrate and socially interact with other members of this community. Well before my first admission I had been a very popular guy but it seemed that at this point there weren't an awful lot of members of the community, including my old associates that wanted to interact with me. My old school crowd were getting on with their careers, forming relationships and getting on with any number of other things that young people do when getting to grips with adult life. I simply didn't see them at that time except the one or two that I ran into by chance as they were at the hospital for other reasons. Even in such chance encounters I had to speak first. I appreciated living in the lodge, where I had gone to re-integrate into the community, as an improvement; however, most of the people I was socially interacting with were still patients from the ward who had come to visit us. One such visitor was the ward's self professed clairvoyant who had the foresight to see that she could more easily profit from her mystic powers beyond the watchful gaze of the ward staff. Well that was one prediction she got right and she was definitely one of the ward survivors. From the perspective of my housemate and myself her colourful personality brightened what could have otherwise been our dismal lives enough to be considered adequate rent for all the time she spent in our abode.

I had been somewhat institutionalised from my time on the wards and although my stay on the lodge did result in forcing me to relearn some of my living skills and opened up a wider range of social opportunities, it was far from immediate independence. My ever present yearning for social contact outside the mental health services was never even nearly met during this period. The lodge experience was very positive on the whole, an important stepping stone to freedom, however, this was not an immediate solution to most things and this young man's overwhelming hungry desires to explore the adult world knew no patience. Often I would gaze through the window, looking at the bus stop, hoping that someone I knew would step off the bus and they would be coming to see me. This never happened. My family were my only visitors from outside the mental health services community and they always came by car. They were non-judgemental, always gave their love, even attended my appointments with my psychiatrist and I always looked forward to their visits with great enthusiasm. Samantha, my youngest sister would help me out with cooking and chores even though she was still at school and my middle sister, Cheryl, would invite me to her house for Sunday lunch. Not only were Cheryl's Sunday dinners legendary but my visits to her house gave me a very homely feel, as I was with family and this was a great contrast to the hospital grounds. My grandparents always welcomed me to their house which also helped me escape the hospital grounds for a time and be in a more home-like environment, I had a couple of uncles who would take me for walks and my brother Dave would take me to play snooker and pool. Dave and I would also lift weights together in his own makeshift gym in his house. In terms of family last but certainly not least I could visit my mother who would buy me all sorts of useful items from clothing to things for my house; you name it from a wall clock to all sorts of kitchen equipment. When it came to friends although almost all of them had pretty much disappeared there were still a very small number that would welcome my visits, including my life-long friend Julie.

My father and Marina, my eldest sister, were particularly regular attendees of my appointments with my psychiatrist despite the fact that they had busy lives. It still means something to me today that they were ready to either drop other commitments or somehow otherwise squeeze me into their hectic schedules. They never gave up on me no matter how dark things seemed and what would have become of me without this support could be a horror beyond my imagination. Their presence at these appointments with my psychiatrist was of an enormous value. As I had been an inpatient and was still a day patient my appointments would be "ward round" appointments. A "ward round" appointment involves not only a patient's psychiatrist seeing them but all the staff involved in their rehabilitative care that can possibly be present. This can be daunting and overwhelming, particularly if they have an agenda that is unpalatable to the patient. The feeling can be that the staff are all against the patient, ganging up on them to impose their will and all thinking they know best because of their professional experience with additional problematic possibilities of professional egos complicating issues. The fact that a patient might know themselves better than anyone else is often little considered, especially if the patient is in no fit state to be assertive or if anything from the patient's history can be used to suggest that they are irresponsible and decisions have to be made for them. Well whatever the rights and wrongs of these ideas it is usually better for the patient if they have the support of loving family members present at these meetings.

This would allow them to have a more comfortable experience of these clinical interviews, so that they might have the confidence to be better self-advocates and so the family members, who also usually know the individual concerned better than the staff, can have their input too. A simple technique used in diplomacy is to have as many diplomats as possible arguing for your cause, at any one debate, and try to outnumber the opposition wherever possible as weight of numbers is very powerful. Needless to say if many staff members wish to impose something unwelcome on an isolated patient their ability to resist is somewhat limited and unfortunately I have to report that the unpleasant effects of stigma can be seen and felt in these very appointments. I do not wish to criticise all mental health staff here by any means as even at this time I met many extremely responsible professionals but still encountered the attitude that as I was just someone who was mentally ill, my opinion could not possibly be worth as much as theirs, and it was even ridiculous to consider that it might. My co-author also points out that he has witnessed the same phenomena and even very responsible mental health staff, who are otherwise a credit to the service, can unwittingly lapse into this behaviour when perhaps tired, stressed and want their own way. The purpose of these criticisms is not to downgrade the staff, as their job is very difficult and at times bordering on the impossible, but more to point out how lapses in their usual high standards are experienced by the unfortunate patient. This book does say more about the negative behaviours of the staff than the positive behaviours as it is about patient experience and pain can be an intense experience lasting long in the memory, however, it does not seek to create a false impression of the staff being more bad than good as this was not the case overall and there were some real heroes amongst them. Simply getting back to the point in most cases having family present at ward rounds creates a better balance and can sometimes even give more useful information to the staff in more fortunate situations when everyone is on the same side.

During my period in the lodge I never had a community worker to facilitate my re-integration into the community and the mental health services staff that I did have contact with were mostly ward staff, giving me the feel that I hadn't put much distance between the wards and myself. I am not alone when I suspect that the ward staff were also institutionalised to some extent by the whole machine of the mental health system, particularly in bygone days when rules surrounding routines were a little stricter, and one really needed to be independent of them to truly escape. The lodge did not represent freedom itself but I got a taste of it and a better idea of what it could be really like. Remember as I had been ill since the age of 16, I had never truly experienced the liberty that comes with adulthood.

## Chapter 5: A human being with problems rather than a problem human being

At my last ward round appointment with my psychiatrist, whilst living in the lodge, it was decided that I was well enough to take the next step towards full integration into the community. I liked this psychiatrist very much and she was ready to give me a chance. The next step was that I was to go to live in a house owned by a housing association and whilst there I was to be supported by the charity "Mind". A charge nurse, that was later to become a friend, showed me around the place and straight away I decided that I liked it. He did not rush me and even seemed to share my enthusiasm. There were many people looking at this one and out of those who wanted it the most suitable two candidates to live there had to be chosen. I was very pleased to be chosen to be one but the competition might not have been too strong as no one else was chosen to live there with me. This house was a two up two down about a mile out of Rotherham town centre and quite badly in need of decorating. Thankfully the "Back-to-Work group" helped me out, just as I had helped many others previously with their re-integrative community ventures.

After being at this new residence for a few months I was asked how I felt about someone sharing with me. The mental health services staff had a particular guy in mind. I had met him previously and he was ok, however, he was not my ideal housemate. I am certainly not the kind of bloke that has ever obsessively gone around my home with a frilly apron on and a feather duster in hand, however, I have always been tidy and keen on hygiene as I was brought up that way. This gentleman was not of such a disposition and it was blatantly obvious from his dishevelled appearance and nickname that this was the case. Aside from the domestic horror of sharing with such a man was the very apparent issue to me that should he live with me I would be marked, everyone would know that there was something different about me (or something wrong with me as folk phrase it) and the full force of the stigma would have followed me out of the hospital allowing me practically no chance to evade it.

Whilst in this neighbourhood people would say hello, as they knew nothing of my past, however, there was a downside to this as there I was on the estate knowing no one and not knowing how to get to know people. In addition to this was the fear that someone would find out about me and word would spread to everyone living around me: I couldn't go through that again. I had a sense of freedom being out, physically free in the community but I was a prisoner in my mind. Whenever I chose I could walk anywhere I wanted but I could not afford to share what I had been through with anyone that did not already know. My mind, heart and soul were bursting to cry out and shout out about my ordeal in the hope that someone would understand and relieve my pain. Frustration and bitter loneliness were to become a way of life for some time to come.

**Stigma: Worse than Psychosis**

Institutionalisation had already got a hold on me and while in the midst of my free but cold life back in the community, I was very powerfully drawn back to the comfort zone of the mental health services. I frequently attended the carwash but would tell people that I was working at the hospital as if I was a conventional employee. At that time I also had other involvements with the mental health services but kept all my contact with them apart from my community life, as though I were living some sort of secret double life. Gradually the euphoria of the independence wore thin as I was feeling increasingly lonely, lost, isolated and cut-off from the rest of the human race. Though my family were great and they could not be any better than they had been while in hospital, the only real difference in social contact terms was that I was now largely cut-off from the people I knew in hospital, from whom I did not have to hide my circumstances from.

In the world I grew up in it certainly was not acceptable for a man, no matter how young, to talk about his feelings. There and then I was desperate to talk about mine. Had I done so to anyone I probably would have very quickly learned why everyone else wasn't doing it as the consequences would probably have been so great. However, if I had the right outlet, the right person or people to talk to it would definitely have been the right thing to do and would have helped enormously. I sometimes wonder if many a male suicide victim has fallen into this macho male behaviour code trap when just finding the right, safe situation in which to

talk would have led to an infinitely better outcome. It is almost certain that my family would have been there to lend a sympathetic ear had I approached them, however, I was very aware of the fact that they were weighed down with many troubles of their own at that time and felt that I had already burdened them enough. Unfortunately at the time I was experiencing all this, the culture of counselling that seems so prevalent today almost didn't exist. Thankfully this is an area in which the mental health services have improved much and in the line of my work I meet many young men, often tough kids too, who need to talk and benefit from it. It took me quite some years to realise that being able to talk about your feelings is a strength and not a weakness; obviously one has to find the appropriate situation in which to do so but once found it may massively change your world for the better.

During this period I developed great social anxieties about being recognised as being mentally ill and these anxieties limited my movements and freedom as there were certain places I just could not go, as it was almost inevitable that I would be known and there would be trouble. I wish to state here that this was definitely not paranoia or even a phobia but was very real fear of a very real problem. I had a reputation around town from my earlier exploits and so was very well known and of those who did not know of me many wanted to. I had problems walking into pubs many times but one particular time sticks in my memory. A group of guys recognised me, jeering at me, with one shouting "what's it like in the nut-house?" Although I was not physically afraid of them I just walked away and this was largely in case an argument led to a fight. People including the authorities, might believe I had initiated the violence as I was mentally ill and that I was not safe to be out loose in the community.

However, I did not simply give up on community interaction as one day I had gone into town and when I saw a young woman, who was still older than me, and her shopping bag burst open I helped her pick her shopping up. I soon found myself in a relationship with her and discovering that she had worked as a psychiatric nurse previously helped with my confidence tremendously. Prior to this I had struggled for female attention off women who were not psychiatric patients themselves and then suddenly I had an ex-psychiatric nurse for a partner. This made me feel that I had covered some ground and that I could be accepted in the community. Better still was the fact that this was the beginning of my first ever serious relationship which is obviously an important milestone in anyone's adult life and particularly significant to me as I seemed to be waiting forever to start it. Amongst the many delights and benefits of this new experience was the fact that for the first time in four years, I found myself sat at a family table on a regular basis. This amazing woman was a totally positive influence on me and saw me as a human being with problems rather than a problem human being.

Unbeknown to me she had been a serious drinker but had moderated it considerably upon meeting me. We would go out socialising around the town centre but would run into some of her old fellow serious drinking associates. Many of these people were very decent folk who had simply slipped into their way of life through a variety of circumstances and I found that amongst such company I was more accepted than I was in non-hard-drinking spheres of society that were supposedly more respectable. This was my social integration amongst people who were prepared to accept me and although I realised these people we seemed to be mixing amongst lived very chaotic lifestyles, including some of them fighting a lot and some being very promiscuous, it took a young Jason Tune a long time to realise that these new associates were not really typical adult members of the community.

As I had only ever really lived in the community properly before as a child, I had little sense of what normal adult behaviour was like and although I had some idea that these people could be a little wild in their ways, I really didn't realise or fully appreciate what kind of people I was mixing with. Even when I recognised a few faces from the psychiatric ward the penny still didn't drop, not because I was stupid or anything but because I was pre-occupied by having a better time than I had had for ages and because I just didn't realise there was a penny there to drop. Obviously I had heard the term "alcoholic" before but in my youthful naïvety I simply thought that an alcoholic was someone who simply drank quite a bit more than most and had no idea of the impact on their lifestyle and the sub-culture that many of them find themselves involved in. There was I knowing nothing about this strange, but often colourful, species of hominid and I was smack bang in the middle of their scene.

One reason I that I became immersed in this world so rapidly, without the alarm bells going off, had been the lack of prejudicial barriers, relative to other social spheres, keeping me out and so I had felt welcome. Even in this world, however, I hadn't completely escaped the evils of being stigmatised. I recall one occasion when upon entering a town hostelry with my new love one of the clientele, who knew my lady friend, pointed at the side of her own head and said "he's been up 'ere 'e 'as", which was her way of denouncing me as some kind of monster and warning my girlfriend to stay away from me as I was mad. I don't know about mad but I was quite upset. Actually I was hurt and it was a threat to my new found happiness. My girlfriend had helped me radically change my life for the better and to lose her through something like this would have totally destroyed me. In this particular incidence my slanderer and one of her daughters became significantly mentally ill themselves. This kind of irony has not been unusual throughout my life for example, also around this time, two guys in a gang that were taunting me in a busy town pub, whilst I was on my own, were shouting out "what's it like in nuthouse?" Both these men also became significantly mentally ill themselves and if I wished I could list many other examples. Some of theses people could be said to be obnoxious but a lot of it came from ignorance and sometimes fear. If someone will taunt another person about having a mental illness, when they are prone to such an ailment themselves, just not yet diagnosed, then it is likely that they have little knowledge of what mental illness actually is. It had taken a massive effort to make the degree of recovery I had by this point and people identifying me as someone who had been a psychiatric patient was threatening my moral, my chances of being accepted out in the community and my life chances. It was bad enough living with the daily risk of abuse from an ill informed community but when individuals who were more or less in the same boat were joining in things could seem ridiculous and overwhelmingly hopeless.

It was also difficult not to be a sitting duck to such abuse. If one has a psychiatric record that indicates one has been violent in the past it becomes very dangerous to be involved in any altercation in the community. This is particularly relevant for people who have had recent hospital admissions as there is a tendency for the authorities to put the mentally ill person back in hospital, sectioning them under the Mental Health Act, regardless of who started the fight. The authorities do make some effort to make the right decision, having psychiatric assessments conducted, but their tendency to err on the side of caution still leaves the psychiatric patient vulnerable as there are many trouble causing wide boys who know the score and how to exploit it.

Within a few months my girlfriend was slipping back into her old habits and as I desired family life her lifestyle was not suiting me. She was physically attractive and attracted a lot of attention in the pubs we frequented and social circles we mixed in. Many of these men were making passes at her so overtly that it brought me into conflict with them or were even downgrading me in front of her. Sometimes the men would annoy her so much that she would want me to do something about it. In the state I was in I really didn't need this kind of stress and these sorts of problems could occur at any point whilst in the pubs she liked and she liked to spend so much of her time in these pubs. She didn't seem to have any empathy about how unpleasant it was to constantly have to play this protective role and she did nothing to reduce the incidence of me having to do this. It was obvious she did not want to change her habits and her habits destroyed the pleasure of the relationship to the point that after about nine months I simply walked away, with no hard feelings and we remained friends afterwards but the relationship had definitely ended.

## Chapter 6: Enter the drug scene

After my first serious relationship had ended I found myself living back at my house in the community full-time and at about this time I bumped into my slightly older cousin Tex, who had recently split up with his girlfriend too. Soon he was staying with me and there we were two young single guys with an appetite to explore the adult world, which was still fairly new to each of us, with an abundance of virgin territory to explore and no concept of how many life hardened veterans there were out there waiting to exploit such as us. We weren't about to disappoint them. It was next to no time before we brought two young ladies back to my house; they were soon rolling up cannabis joints and succeeding in convincing us how harmless the drug was. I had briefly smoked tiny quantities of cannabis before in my early teens but had been very wary of it as then I saw it as a scary drug, I had did not smoke much more and had just tried it out of curiosity. Making things fairer we at least managed to convince them that sharing our beds was harmless too, however, our bedroom antics never did them any harm but this night represented the beginning of the slippery slope into the drug scene for me.

Previously my father had kicked out an associate that had being staying with me, who had been a heroin user, I had never been involved in drug use with him. Soon I was smoking cannabis regularly and although it never impacted significantly upon my mental health the long-term effects of cannabis on a person's mind vary tremendously between individuals. These effects are influenced by many factors some of which are known and some which remain a mystery but there is now a large body of evidence to indicate that this substance can really harm some users whilst leaving others relatively unaffected. My co-author has a few comments to make regarding this phenomenon in the next chapter which he writes alone.

## Chapter 7: Cannabis can't harm you it's all a government conspiracy!

This chapter was largely written in response to the growing acceptance of the notion of the dual diagnosis of mental illness and substance misuse, to communicate that amphetamines are not the only culprit and to illustrate the stigma related complications that may affect the afflicted individual.

Ok so how did it begin? Well once upon a time in a land of not so far away, there lived a teenager who had never used drugs before but was suffering anxiety and depression as a result of dire circumstances. Regular binge drinking had begun for him at fourteen which today would probably be considered normal, but back in the days of mullet hairstyles and cheesy music it was a little early. As well as the allure that alcohol has for all of such age there was the additional appeal in that it provided an escape anesthetising his personal pain. At seventeen he was introduced to cannabis, now some would consider such a lad a late starter these days, but back then when enormous shoulder pads were all the rage it was younger than most; or at least in my town it was. Now this young fellow had been curious about cannabis, had been led to believe it was much safer than other drugs to the point it could be danger free and so would have probably tried it anyway, however, his extreme need for an escape made him far more susceptible to desire for regular use and being sucked into the drug social scene that went with it. Ok now I'm sure it doesn't take a genius to work out that this naïve young plonker was me.

Well there I found myself getting further involved with other regular cannabis users slowly absorbing the values and gradually adopting an appearance of a fairly typical cannabis smoker of the time. That is to say the sort of appearance that instantly gave the police a good idea what I was up to. The depression I was suffering from at the time was actually rather serious and had become noticeable to some, but surrounded by cannabis users it was easy to mask as being stoned or straight when not used to it. To people outside drug using circles the combination of the way I came across with my depressed, anxious and slightly agoraphobic personality combined with my appearance was beginning to bring the weight of stigma down upon my head.

Not long after turning eighteen I found myself homeless. I soon found myself living in a house with two relatively new found friends and an army of cat flees but I won't digress about that unpleasant experience. The house belonged to the boyfriend of the mother of the friend I had most recently met out of the two of them. This friend was more just an acquaintance at that time although I was soon to see him as a genuine friend. He probably found my gratitude for giving me somewhere to live, as he was more or less in charge of the house, a little overwhelming but I had experienced a terrible time and was hoping my worst problems were solved. Nothing could have been further from the truth and I had possibly landed in one of the worst places I could as things turned out. This was not in any way because they were drug crazed monsters in fact they were not; they were little older than I and although they might deny it to this day they were easily as naïve. The problem lay in the fact that they had a massive overwhelming enthusiasm for drugs, in particular cannabis and it was impossible not to find this contagious. Soon a heavily depressed 18 year old was stoned day in day out and pinning all his future happiness on drugs and certainly using them to cope with the here and now. It started out as just cannabis use but….

Laugh? Yeah course I laughed, I laughed my nuts off like I'd never laughed so much ever before in my life the day that someone said to me "cannabis use can lead to other drugs" and I did not laugh alone. So many people I know have laughed at this too and often whilst I have been there to witness it and so if it is so funny to so many people then surely the people who say it must be being so ridiculous? It took me a lot of years, and years that I was never guaranteed to make it through to become fully enlightened about exactly who was being ridiculous.

Due to general adolescent power politics, I soon found myself leaving this humble abode to move on to an even more humble abode still living with similar people. A couple more address changes and lots of drugs later I found myself living in a badly rundown house, on my own or rather sort of alone; the house was also used as a rather unconventional taxi base. At least I rented this place legitimately and was officially no longer homeless. By this time, several months after first becoming homeless, my appearance had altered considerably as I had now got very thick, long hair; most of the time was sporting an untrimmed beard, was matchstick thin, wore falling to bits jeans, worn-out footwear and an army surplus jacket which I slept in wherever I lost consciousness when I didn't make it home.

Around this time most of my friends I had made in Rotherham had left, many to go to universities or simply seek adventure and/or work in other parts of the country. I was socially quite isolated, my depression and anxiety levels were appallingly bad and this made it very hard to do my studies as I had resumed my attempt to gain A Levels at the town centre college. This was very stressful for me as passing my A Levels and going to a university was the only route of escape from my miserable and impoverished circumstances that I could envisage. I was not just lonely for general company but I also badly wanted a girlfriend, so badly in fact that it must have put most young ladies off not to mention that my appearance, lifestyle and general psychological state were not in line with most girl's vision of prince charming. To boot in my despair my negative thinking was such that even when the occasional attractive young lady was attracted to me, my mind refused to believe it.

I had chosen Rotherham to be the town I would move to because of all my newfound friends and associates, however, after living there for less than a year I found myself being quite lonely. Many of my peers had moved on to universities and many folk I knew simply moved to other towns as there was little work in Rotherham. As for most of the rest of my associates, I had realised many of them were excessively involved in crime other than recreational drug use for my comfort and I distanced myself from them or I had fallen out with them. Unfortunately I lost out on the company of some of them for a reason far sadder than that; the fact that they wanted to spend most of their time involved in healthy activities of the kind that help an adolescent in their development whereas I wanted to be constantly stoned. This simply meant that we didn't have enough in common any more to find each other's company stimulating.

Soon I stumbled across a clique of people, the individuals of which I had mostly not met before and found that they were equally enthusiastic about travelling down the path of self destruction as I was. They were a sort of more extreme sub group of the wider drug using circles I had been moving in. More extreme in that they regarded themselves as even more outside conventional society and more extreme in that they were pressing the self-destruct button that bit harder.

There were many things that I was uneasy about when it came to spending time with these people. One being that that a couple of them were people I had previously tried to avoid because of their criminal activities, but I had to accept them or lose the whole group and face social isolation. I did not know them well but was dependent on them in very disempowering circumstances. Well at least I had people to take drugs with.

Being dependent on this group of people, that although not necessarily bad, made me feel very uncomfortable. The combination of the stress I was under because of the pain of what had happened in my past (a harrowing later childhood), the stress of sheer poverty, the stress of having to succeed at my studies as the only way to escape my circumstances, the stress of studying itself whilst ill with severe depression and anxiety and the stress of being dependent on a group of people that I was actually very uncomfortable with for deliverance from isolation all mounted up and stress is a trigger for psychosis. So what did I do to relieve this stress? I smoked large amounts of cannabis, another known trigger for psychosis though not known so much at the time.

I had experienced some paranoia and strange perceptions whilst smoking cannabis but as most people do it was difficult to determine whether I was experiencing more than most other people, especially as everyone around me would keep telling me it was normal and cannabis was totally safe. In contrast to this, I have never had any paranoia whilst under the influence of magic mushrooms or LSD which most people on the drug scene would insist were more likely to induce it. As

I seemed to be controlling the magic mushrooms and LSD perfectly it seemed logical to assume that what I experienced on cannabis was normal.

Many people on the drugs scene had insisted that after an LSD or magic mushroom experience was mostly over, it was best to smoke cannabis to "come down". They would often insist this protected against having a bad experience. I had always ignored this and never had a bad time coming down from these drugs. However, this new crowd I was spending time with insisted on this practice and they were the ones I was taking magic mushrooms with in the autumn of that year. In the weeks prior to this I had been becoming paranoid on cannabis significantly more often than usual, with bizarre thinking and perceptions involved. It would have been wise to interpret these as warning signs but my need for an escape combined with my need to smoke it to fit in with everyone I knew meant quitting was virtually out of the question.

The first time I recall using cannabis specifically to come down off a magic mushroom trip I remember a tremendously physically pleasant sensations and the world around me changing markedly; I was more intoxicated than when peaking from the magic mushrooms themselves. It felt good, however, I had even then an intuitive suspicion that my mind had altered that bit too much and that the boat had been pushed out too far to get back to shore. At that time I did not care much and just carried on feeling good. I had not returned to normal before the next magic mushroom experience in which, again, I used cannabis to come down and this left me even further from the safe and familiar shores of reality.

Following a succession of similar experiences my behaviour became a little more eccentric and bizarre, reflecting my mental state and it was very conspicuous to the group I was spending time with. Things came to a head one evening when, although unsure if magic mushrooms were involved at the time, copious quantities of cannabis were and the group definitely seemed to be working together playing some sort of cryptic, bizarre mind game with me. Eventually I felt I was loosing control over my mind and feared for my safety in the house I was in and quickly made for the door. After my quick, seemingly strange to this group, exit I decided no more drugs or at least not until I returned to my normal state. Even now, twenty years on, I have not properly returned to that normal state, oh well, fingers crossed maybe in another twenty years eh?

"Caught with my pants down? I got caught with my pants down by the Martians on the f***ing Moon man!" Was my immediate response to Jason when he was talking about there being nothing like one's first experience of drug induced psychosis and asked if I was caught with my pants down the first time that drugs made me ill.

Let me now describe my subjective experience of the progression of the onset of my experience of first episode psychosis as best as I remember it. Many days passed during which I barely slept and sleep deprivation alone can initiate psychosis. During this period I started to believe I had magical powers, and had realised all sorts of strange things were going on around me. I came to believe that prior to this period I had been living life with blinkers on and I had suddenly come to see reality but there were still a few things I did not understand and there was some confusion in my world. Soon I was due to see my psychiatrist and I believed they would reveal to me the final secrets of the universe and all the pieces would fall into place. To my surprise she did not know what I was talking about and got between me and the door when I tried to leave, telling me I was in for a stay on the psychiatric ward.

Whilst in hospital at first I was on a manic high but was paranoid at the same time. I had drifted into a kind of paranoid fantasy world. Many of my ideas had a supernatural theme usually involving religion, most seemed to have been attempts to explain the world I was in and did not understand.

I thought I had reached some degree of enlightenment and had started to see the real world for the first time and all the people who attained this insight gained magical powers, but I was having trouble using mine possibly because I had not achieved full enlightenment. I thought there were hidden messages in some people's conversations and I had to decipher what they meant in order to fully attain this higher state of consciousness.

At first I had no idea that I was ill and one point thought the hospital was a place where such knowing people went to; perhaps finely tune their magical powers though I did have different theories about what the hospital was. Similarly I had lots of theories about what the law was and after absconding from the hospital and being found, I was threatened with being detained on a Home Office section, but had little idea of what that really meant, just more supernatural theories. These ideas may simply make me seem stupid, well, from my perspective at least part of the experience seemed to involve my mind racing so much that I did not have time to rationally analyse my vast number of rapidly generated thoughts the way I had previously and I was overwhelmed.

Soon I was in great distress through not knowing what was going on around me and the anxiety was intensely painful. I was desperate to make sense of what was going on and to relieve my anxiety. During this time I entertained many bizarre theories about what was going on around me and in the world: all were attempts to make sense of my situation and the world generally.

The psychiatrists were prescribing me all sorts of drugs at this time. The people I had been doing illegal drugs with were telling me not to take the psychiatrist's drugs, that they were bad for me and some of these people even said that what I needed was more cannabis to chill my mind out. In the state I was in, I did not appreciate what medical qualifications were worth and did not see the psychiatrists who were prescribing drugs as any wiser than illicit drug users who recommended taking illegal drugs.

Unfortunately many of the psychiatrist's drugs were harming me. I was having intensely bad reactions to them but was unable to communicate this successfully to the nursing staff and all I could do was to try to refuse them. This led to the nursing staff putting what seemed like intense pressure on me to take these drugs that were causing me more pain. This made it harder to believe the psychiatrists and see the drug users as being wrong. What seemed like intense pressure was probably in fact only mild but in my hyper-sensitive state I experienced it that way.

Thankfully, eventually, it was realised that the medication was not working and I was offered Electro-Convulsive-Therapy. My drug using friends were saying 'don't have it' and 'they want to fry your brain'. They really saw it that way. I was afraid of the idea but I was desperate and so agreed to have it.

I was so lucky. I responded to it straight away and it was truly like a miracle cure. Pretty much straight away, I realised I was just in a hospital and my ideas of magical goings on had almost disappeared. Largely I could say I had gone from being insane to being sane again.

The psychiatrist said that I had had a Schizophreniform reaction, which is largely experiencing some schizophrenic symptoms for a period of time, a few weeks, triggered off by illicit drug use or stress. After this I was considered to be mostly a sufferer of just depression and anxiety. However some symptoms lingered on although lessened in severity, those being de-realisation, which is the world looking and feeling somehow unreal, paranoia but to a lesser extent and hearing things.

I have never heard voices telling me to do things, but I would hear people discussing me everywhere I went. If people were talking in the distance away from me I would hear them discussing me, knowing great details about me even if I had never seen them before.

My drug-taking friends persuaded me that cannabis was not strong enough to have caused my illness and that it was probably caused by the magic mushrooms and LSD, which seem to be stronger drugs. It was to be years later that I would find out, partly through a psychiatrist and partly through my own reading, that although cannabis is less intoxicating than magic mushrooms or LSD, it was the most likely of the drugs to have caused my schizophrenic symptoms because of its biochemical action in the brain. It had also felt like it was the cannabis making me ill at the time and in such a clear way that the connection should have been obvious. However, an army of enthusiastic cannabis smokers around me, that absolutely refused to believe anything negative about their revered drug, easily overpowered my mind (which was rather malleable at the time) and convinced me that it was the other drugs that had not agreed with me. Unfortunately I did not know this at the time. I got out of hospital and resumed smoking it, largely because life was not good enough and I needed an escape.

Within less than twelve months I realised cannabis was causing me to be paranoid. It would bring on paranoia at the time I smoked it, which is common, but I wouldn't quite return to normal afterwards when the cannabis should have wore off and so gradually my straight state was becoming more and more paranoid. Because of this deterioration I stopped using it. I carried on hearing people talking about me and it was impossible not to respond to it in some ways and it affected how I behaved towards people that I thought had said things about me. I knew at least some of it was unreal but deciding what was and what was not was difficult because sometimes people genuinely can discuss one while one is within hearing distance. This problem was intense and caused me much anxiety. It was worse at times when stressful things were going on in my life but the long term picture seemed to be that things were getting better.

I did various college courses, lost a sponsorship through my illness, although my sponsors never knew what was wrong, held down a job for two years despite being ill and again lost the job through my illness although I never let the employer know I was ill. Then I decided to get more qualifications so I could do a university degree. I wanted to study psychology partly because I still thought I could one day be well and have a career and partly because I wanted to help myself.

In 1994 around Christmas time, whilst studying for more A Levels, I had a major relapse. This time I had not been taking drugs or even had a drink for about four months leading up to this episode but stress may have been the trigger. The problem of hearing people talking about me became intense again and I had other paranoid delusions. I found myself with the memories of scores of abusive phone calls having been made to me by people who had known me all through my past, but I was not sure when these phone calls had been made. In my mind hundreds of people from my past were all working together in one conspiracy and had been frequently phoning me with threats and abuse. One thing I thought some of them were trying to achieve was to get me to commit suicide.

This time I was given different medication that calmed me down but the memories were still clear. Even to this day I wonder if some of the calls were real. The medication helped me over the crisis and I was less ill over the next four years or so in which time I went to a university and gained a degree in psychology. The things I had learned helped a lot and enabled me to see my situation more clearly. Soon after I graduated I began preparing for a PhD but I realised I would have to shelve my plans because I was too ill. I have probably experienced no significant true paranoia since my Christmas 1994 relapse although for many years I remained highly susceptible to anxiety provoking thoughts and stress. In the millennium year I was extremely ill for some weeks, however, it was a response to genuine stressful events and so could more be simply understood as anxiety.

Right from making the connection between my ill health and cannabis, around the beginning of autumn 1990, I realised that in order to minimise my illness I had to absolutely avoid this drug and drugs generally and to maximise my chances of doing this I had to escape the influence of people encouraging me to take such substances. It would be many years later that I became aware of the full strength of this connection, however, it was at this time I realised the need to extricate myself from the drugs scene.

Leaving a drug sub-culture behind, something that both Jason and myself had been forced to do simply for the sake of survival, involved a leap into the unknown and was a fearful journey into a world of near social isolation. It doesn't take a long period of regular drug use for some people to find themselves moving only in circles in which practically everyone else is a drug user and the ability to relate well to non-drug users can fade fast. One even acquires altered use of language that seems outlandish outside those circles, which along with altered dress style adds to the alienation from the rest of society. Giving up a drug often involves leaving almost everyone that you know, or in extreme unfortunate circumstances everyone, behind and starting again. This is difficult as the drug sub-culture might have caused a person to have a major problem relating to non-drug users and may even distrust them. Adding to this problem of making new friends is the fact that people normally make friends by meeting them through other friends, but if you have none it can be difficult to get the ball rolling. To further the problem if one also has a reputation for having used drugs it can be even harder to establish a cleaner living social circle and if one is also known to have had mental health issues (whether still ill or recovered) the stigma that accompanies this makes the task no easier. When thinking about this it is worth bearing in mind that any individual in this position on such a social quest is likely to be devoid of confidence, self esteem and even be depressed: people like to befriend confident, strong people who value themselves and are fun to be around.

People often casually use phrases relating to how strong they or someone else is as a person. Well let me tell you that a totally socially isolated individual has no strength at all, because a human simply can't function that way and a person's apparent strength is mostly just an illusion reflecting the degree to which they have had the right human relationships throughout their lives, both in the past and present, to foster feelings of security. This experience of an adult having to socially start again can be every bit as scary as it is for a child venturing into a playground for the first time. A person's mental health is dependent on them having an adequate basic social network and failure to acquire it or keep it results in failure to function and normally great psychological pain too. There are no options here as success has to be achieved.

The whole business for me was, although necessary, still in some ways rather sad. The drug users I knew were not the frothing at the mouth monsters that perhaps some folk who had never experimented with such substances might think they were. Today illicit drug use is so widespread that very few people are so naïve as to see users that way as almost everyone knows some, however, I am still mostly referring to the time around 1990 when the people on my drugs scene could get a lot of abuse from non-drug-users and this abuse was usually highly inappropriate. Many of the people I knew saw themselves as hippies and genuinely had philosophies that were centred on love and peace: these people were much nicer and possibly better members of society than most of the clean-cut individuals I knew. Still if you tried telling them that cannabis could be harmful they would get very upset and sometimes angry as their subculture was very oriented around the idea that cannabis could do no evil: it was often said that the government claimed it was harmful and didn't want people smoking it because they couldn't tax it. The other people that had been on this drug scene were a mix of good and bad just like any other group in society and I would miss many of them but as fond of them as I was, their influence was harmful to me and I had to distance myself from them.

## Stigma: Worse than Psychosis

All through these years of mental ill health, I have been plagued by the stigma attached to it having had a multitude of bad experiences as a result. The degree of my illness and the way it impacted on my life meant that much of the time it was not possible to hide it and sometimes explanations for my behaviour were or seemed necessary. When first having become ill and most of my associates were still drug users it was best to stress how big a part my drug use played in my illness, as it was deemed more acceptable to go over the edge with drugs than simply be mentally ill. Even so there remained the problem that there would still be criticism for not being able to handle the drug as there seemed to be little understanding, amongst my circle, of how the biochemistry of an individual's brain might not be suited to certain drugs. Most of these people seemed to think everything related to whether someone was wise enough or "together" enough to cope with a drug as though everything depended on a person's personality. This meant I still had inferior status, in the eyes of many, to those who had not become ill.

Additionally I had to go along with the idea that it was drugs other than cannabis that had harmed me as should I suggest that cannabis had the slightest capacity to do harm, I would not be able to bear the weight of criticism. Once outside the drug using circles it really was a tricky business because to simply be seen to have become mentally ill without giving a rational explanation did nothing for one's prestige, however, amongst some the use of illicit drugs carries a greater stigma. If anyone did not like me or any group wished to make sport of me whatever I would say to minimise the danger would result in me being judged the worse; it was all simply a catch-22 situation that I would be repeatedly caught in.

Having done the right things to stay away from drugs over the years and having made many other lifestyle alterations too, I have managed to gradually improve my health to bearable levels. This has meant it has become more difficult for anyone to detect any problem; there are now fewer occasions upon which I find myself in a position whereby I feel it is necessary to disclose my illness and as a result I suffer less from the associated stigma. The long, disciplined, narrow-path journey to better health and liberation from this stigma has only just brought me to having an acceptable quality of life shortly prior to co-writing this book. In fact I've only just managed to finally crawl out of hell, so recently that my arse is still smouldering!

## Chapter 8: Speed Freak

My cousin Tex only stayed at my house for a short while and after he left I soon felt isolated and lonely. Even in hospital I was used to having many people around and almost always had someone to talk to. This fuelled a need for escapism and one day going out to score cannabis, I scored the biggest own goal of my life. I had gone looking for cannabis and unfortunately, as there had been many drug busts in the area, there was a dope famine. In my search, I bumped into a couple of older associates from the estate upon which I had been brought up. They had a mission of their own, which was to sell an item of dubious origin, which ultimately met the fate of being swapped for a bag of amphetamine sulphate. It felt great to see a couple of old familiar faces, especially people who did not reject me and combined with my need for escapism and habit of being used to a buzz, I was easily influenced by them when they suggested I try amphetamines.

I was only twenty at the time and although I had been in a fair few scuffles in my short life, I was still very naïve about drugs. I had my underlying mental health problems and additional issues as a relationship had recently ended with someone whom I cared very much about. All in all I was very vulnerable at this time and easily swayed by two older familiar faces, which knew my situation and presented themselves as wise friends, who knew how to help me achieve happiness. Well I guess I was a sitting duck and proof of this was the fact that despite having developed somewhat of a phobia of needles from my days on the acute wards, within next to no time one of them was injecting me with an illegal drug that I knew nothing about. Don't try this at home kids! I know that I am not the only person that this has happened to and many drug users, often wide boys and members of the broader criminal fraternity, target the vulnerable to involve them in their drug use for a multitude of reasons. Such reasons included profiteering and simply wanting more associates to share their interest with. Whilst deliberately trying to bring about the fall of someone, who has not ruined their own life yet out of jealousy and misguidedly thinking, they were doing their victim a favour. The dealing predator still thought the drug enhances people's lives. There are many such predators out there in all sorts of forms and I was such easy prey, but at least I am still around to tell the tale unlike many. Within a very short space of time I was deeply immersed in the drug scene and although only heavily involved for about five years in total, I found myself attending eight drug related funerals.

Although these guys did not physically force me to take the drug, the culmination of factors making me susceptible to their influence virtually made it a forgone conclusion that I would yield to their persuasion. Largely being brought up by my grandparents, who were not armed with the knowledge necessary to warn an adolescent about drugs, had meant I was not prepared for this situation. My circumstances at the time, including isolation, meant that I had no strength to resist the temptations that would seriously challenge any young man such as curiosity, the desire for acceptance and to be one of the lads. Suddenly I was drawn into a world where mentally ill people were accepted and even commonplace. I am sure many other mentally ill people were drawn in out of being vulnerable in a similar manner to myself, but also many people who had no mental health problems prior to drug use developed them as a result. My time spent on the drug scene lead me to observe that many people suffering mental health problems would use drugs as an escape and whatever the order of events, whether the mental illness preceded the drug use or vice versa, it seemed that the two acted like a vicious cycle spiralling downwards. Does it matter which came first the chicken or the egg if they both end up full of salmonella?

Just like the way many people report their first experience of certain drugs my first rush on amphetamine was the best I ever got. High as a kite I was, but never was I able to get that hit again. Just the same as many other drug users, I spent the time immediately following my first use trying to repeat the experience. Like many other drug users, by the time I'd realised I was never going to be able to reach such a high ever again, I was hooked.

This represented another major life and lifestyle change. I had already had a period involved with Rotherham's serious pub drinking mini-subculture within which the doors were pretty much open to people with a mental illness. This had represented a bubble in which to be relatively free from stigma; well the drug scene represented a more extreme version of this. However, although it may be obviously apparent to the reader, whether individuals in the drug scene had mental health problems or not we all carried a stigma in the eyes of most people outside this social sphere. Just as most stigmatised groups tend to be subdivided, illicit drug users in most towns are also. Developing a ravenous appetite for amphetamines lead me to spend the bulk of my time with other serious amphetamine users and dealers that specialised in the retail of this product who were usually partial to their own wares. I would encounter connoisseurs of other noxious substances far more often than members of the non-drug-using community, but they were still mostly on the outskirts of my rather specialised social scene.

The people of this scene met the criteria for being a persecuted minority as amongst other things people who knew very little about us would often hate us, abuse us or at very least view us as being inferior. This led to some degree of strengthening of bonds within the drug using community, as these people sharing common interests needed to pull together for strength and support. In fact at times parts of the drug scene could seem like one big happy family, both from the perspective of one of its members or an outsider looking in. Well that's how it can seem at times when there is a plentiful supply of their drug of choice, that is affordable and of a quality that meets their approval. Now how do you think things are when the supply is poor, everything is expensive, all products adulterated and most people don't even have the money to go and get ripped off? You must have heard the saying "times are hard and friends are few" well multiply that by a thousand and you might be able to picture the drug scene when resources are scarce. The comradeship of the transient good times is sometimes re-kindled for a short while at the odd funeral, but largely one has to look after oneself whilst in a state ill equipped to do so.

Speed Freak, Phet 'ed, and Whizz 'ed were some of the labels used for my cosy little section of the drug scene, with these terms being largely used by all from disapproving outsiders to members of our own fraternity. My absorption into this sub-culture within sub-culture led me away from my treatment. Not just by way of distraction but now I had a circle of associates amongst whom I was not stigmatised and wanting to forget that I had ever been ill, I totally broke off contact with the health services. I thought this would help prevent the stigma following me further through all facets of my life and I gave little consideration to the fact that this decision meant the discontinuation of all forms of treatment. Unwittingly as I made these manoeuvres of rather dubious wisdom, in order to evade the stigma of mental illness, I was inviting another stigma into my life. One deemed to be darker, self-deserving and more sinister in the eyes of many.

Ok so why take these substances when it is common knowledge to so many that they can be so harmful and detrimental to one's quality of life? What one normally hears about after everything has gone wrong, in the cases when the user is still alive and sane enough to tell the tale is how good the early effects once were. One also hears about how good a time they were having and how they were surrounded by fellow users preaching about how the drug is not as dangerous as it is made out to be. Well although I have described the business of the first hit being the best, I have not yet mentioned the fact that, although consecutive hits obey the law of diminishing returns, if one is prepared to increase the dosage one can still achieve a substantial hit for some time before the milk turns sour. Something that users may also speak of, but perhaps with less frequency, is about how much the initial good times were influenced by the drug scene they were part of and their associates, rather than the actual drug itself.

At the time of my initiation into all this, I was far from the only new recruit to the ranks of the amphetamine users. My newfound associates and apparent friends were mostly a combination of new users, very excited about the novelty such as myself and older, more experienced users that were very much survivors on the scene, adept at manipulation and able to exploit the new cannon fodder such as yours truly. The older users that had become casualties were mostly either in graves, too mentally or physically ill to be out in public much or so mad that people would avoid them.

They didn't want much to do with other users as they just wanted to get their drugs, or in happier cases had managed to escape the scene. In summary they were largely out of sight, not there to act as a bad advertisement for amphetamines or warn new victims about them, but had they been, we were having such a good time the message may have had limited impact. Largely speaking the more experienced users we came across were mostly wide-boys who knew how to sell us the good time.

There were no shortage of young women on the amphetamines scene and they often helped the parties go with a bang. Amphetamines make people more uninhibited and sometimes increase a woman's libido. I had enjoyed myself on the Northern Soul scene but this seemed a level above that life, being simply a succession of parties, at least at first. My whole identity had seemingly improved as I was happier to be known as a "druggy" than someone who had mental health problems. What I know now but didn't know then was that many people use drugs and the drugs scene to mask mental health problems. The way it works is that people, who do not want others to know they have mental health problems or even admit it to themselves, will dismiss the symptoms they experience as effects of drugs. This serves the dual role of hiding their mental illness and even often giving them kudos, as anyone taking so much of a drug as to get such effects must be wild and cool which, helps them deny they are ill to others, or even stay in denial about it themselves thus protecting their self image. In certain sections of the drug using community, there are even strong anti-psychiatry philosophies preaching negative propaganda about the mental health services and particularly the effects of drugs often prescribed by psychiatrists. It's true enough that drugs companies can promote a seemingly unrealistic rosy picture about the efficacy of such drugs and the rarity of their side effects; however, the rumours floating around the drugs scene frequently take suspicions about such medications and the intentions of their prescribers to extremes.

The distrust this breeds acts as a further barrier to drug users experiencing psychiatric illness seeking help as, in part, they view their mental phenomena through a philosophical perspective that denies psychiatric knowledge and instead draws on any number of alternative explanations, that often include conspiracy theories of one form or another. How can an individual beat paranoia in a paranoid social environment? Perhaps a large proportion of mentally ill people within these circles that wish to deny their mental illness help feed this fear? I'm sure this fear works well for the profiteering wide-boys on the scene, as if their customers listened to the recommendations of the psychiatrists they would experience their own recession. Still the whole business of masking mental illness with drugs worked quite well for me at first, whilst still getting the highs and I'm sure I am not alone in this.

During this time I kept a considerable distance from my family as, although I was enjoying myself at first, I immediately knew that my family would disapprove and that it could bring great shame on them if people knew that their son was a junkie. I felt I had already brought enough shame on them, taxed their kindness more than I felt comfortable with and the last way I wished to repay this great kindness and support was to stain the family's reputation further. Basically I was limiting contact with my family, at a time when they were the ones that stood the best chance in the world of steering me away from this path of destruction. It was the exact opposite move that I needed to make, but the one that most naïve young fools make when entering such circles; even my co-author says it was that way for him and most folk he knew who fell into the same trap. This is something largely encouraged on the drug scene in which, between them, the other users have a wealth of experience at leading new recruits further in and separating them from people who might warn them thus cutting their life-lines.

Parents and "straights" (people who don't use illegal drugs) are "square" amongst many other things and soon the new drug user, very enthusiastic about their new hobby, wants to talk excitedly about it all the time which of course they can't do to non-users who soon seem so boring not to mention a security risk. Contact with my relatives did not completely end as I occasionally visited them for dinners, but I was deliberately vague in communicating my activities at this time and even kept communication minimal. Many kinds of family functions that previously I would have attended were not even considered on my social agenda, as I felt I had found a new and exhilarating lifestyle, free from the old stigma all be it still a lifestyle I had to be secretive about.

You're mad you are! People would often say to me during this time. Well I didn't know whether they were referring to my psychiatric history, the fact that I had made the decision to be an amphetamine user or the effects of the drug on my mind there and then. My amphetamine fuelled psyche spent much time and energy poring over this point and in each instance of me hearing the remark gauging how to respond to the individual making such an utterance. This experience was frequently extremely uncomfortable and other phenomena were entering my world of drug use that was tipping the balance of benefits to deficits in the direction of reduced quality of life and I personally was threatening to become unbalanced. It wasn't so long before I realised this wonderful new way of living was not so great, the illusion was dissipating and I decided that before my dream life could turn into a nightmare, I would opt out. Soon amphetamine dealers, with high status on the scene, were visiting me trying to sell me the dream again. It was as if vultures were coming to claim me even though I wasn't dead yet.

Ploys to draw me back into amphetamine use included these wide boy dealers attempting to convince me that amphetamine users were an exclusive group of people that had seen through the system and were having an amazing time that ordinary people, who were no more than mugs, could never imagine. They often sold this story to people of the amphetamine scene being full of elitist people who were higher forms of life than the rest of humanity. Much of the time they seemed to believe their own propaganda. Their tactics also included, for both recruiting new users and for re-enticing people they were trying to draw back into the scene, injecting vulnerable people with amphetamines the moment they became susceptible to their spin and doing this swiftly before they changed their minds.

Has anyone seen similar tactics used with any other drugs? Please send answers in on a postcard reader. One of their phenomenally socially damaging tactics, which is much under-reported on, is alienating their recruits/victims from all those who could lead them in another direction and not just family (as already mentioned). The dealers would try to instil a deep distrust and fear of the medical world, the police, the legal system and basically any societal institution, group of individuals or individual that spoke a message contrary to theirs. They did this to do the potential drug user a favour, to enhance their life and help them see the truth; it just so happened that in the process they made an awful lot of money out of it and acquired more people below them in the social order of their sub-culture (people whom they could exert power over).

In my youth and naïvety I knew nothing about psychological addiction. Many people around me, both predators trying to draw me into the scene and others as naïve as me who had also been fooled, kept telling me how amphetamines were not physically addictive and this had been a major selling point to both myself and countless others. However, I still felt totally burnt out, I was not at home surrounded by many of the people around me that were from the criminal fraternity and I knew that if I did not get out of this scene soon I would regress back to the worst state I had ever been in, or possibly worse. The decision was made, my very survival depended upon escaping the scene and that was what I had to do.

## Chapter 9: A stigma free paradise

Desperation for an escape from this false stigma free world had overcome me, along with a myriad of other immediate and non-ignorable salient reasons for getting out and facing the hard facts of my situation head on, with no hiding or pretence. Soon I went through the horrors of amphetamine withdrawals unsupported. This might seem foolish to any sensible reader but I was still influenced by the values and ideals of the hard core amphetamine users sub-culture which, in relation to this situation, were that one should not go forward for help or be identified as such a user by any authorities.

One cannot ordinarily simply stop such an activity or eject oneself from such a scene without replacing it with an alternative way of living. My attempt at a new lifestyle would involve at least attempting to be far more conventional. Almost immediately I found myself sprucing myself up to go out around the Rotherham town centre pub scene. This was quite a leap for me and no less because in the hard-core amphetamine scene within which I had been immersed alcohol was one of the few other drugs that hardly anyone ever used. Soon I was buying a vodka and orange for an attractive young lady in one of these pubs. This was my future wife-to-be and from that day, that period of amphetamine use immediately ended, as my love for her was an infinitely more powerful buzz.

Within a short space of time I was working and more to the point holding the job down and we set up home together. We had got on really well from the beginning and this positively impacted upon my wellbeing, in that I was able to function without medication and needed no contact with the mental health services. In 1988 we got married. By this time I had been working for quite some time as an industrial dismantler and burner and I had managed to catch up with some old non-drug-using friends that became the core of my new social circle. No time was wasted as in late 1988 my son was born. There I was a proud father with everything going right in the world and what was basically a normal life. The days of suffering the stigma of mental illness had largely been left behind, ok so there were some folk who would remember my previous illness but all the evidence that I had ever been ill had dissipated and it was as if it was just some fading memory of a bad dream that I was leaving in the past. Indeed I had seemingly entered some kind of stigma-free paradise that was fast becoming normality.

I scarcely encountered people reminding me of my past and the good life continued. After a while I changed jobs to become a steel erector and worked on two of the largest construction sites the UK has ever had; the largest being the Channel Tunnel. Whilst working on the tunnel, one of my visits back to Rotherham was for my son's christening, during which the vicar included in his speech a snippet about how I was a role model for Rotherham working on this historical construction project and this almost made me as proud as having my family. The next project was to work on high-rise buildings on Canary Wharf. I was earning good money and served an apprenticeship to become a fully qualified steel erector and everything continued to go well. During this period it was apparent that people saw me in a very different light to ever before in my adult life and I was respected, which was of paramount importance as for me the stigma had been worse than the illness itself. However, unfortunately by the end of the summer of 1990, on a weekend visit home, my wife announced to me that she no longer had the feelings for me that she once had and she turned out to be seeing another man, who was supposedly an old friend of mine.

My world shattered leaving me in a heap of devastation and this was just the beginning, as a very messy divorce was to follow, after which I would not get to see my son, then two, for another fourteen years. I had to get solicitors involved in the divorce and I lost contact with my son, I believe, mostly through mental health stigma even though my psychiatric reports, produced in court, were favourable. Work became my escape during this period and involved me doing long hours to evade the pain. Holding my job down was not a problem as it was a positive in my life, however, unfortunately I returned to amphetamine use which was obviously a major negative in my life. Instead of talking to anyone about my situation, I tried to blank out the pain by other means. This was also around the time that my brother took his life and I was emotionally destroyed by this loss and wrapped with guilt. The divorce case and custody battle dragged on and in my emotionally dilapidated state, I found myself actually being influenced by the advice given to me by people on the amphetamine scene who's prime concern was taking as much of my money off me as possible. Prior to this my only close losses had been my grandparents, which had hurt enough, but loosing my younger brother at 24 years old took grief to a whole new level. In addition to the grief was my guilt about not having been able to help him. Trying to negotiate courtroom strategy whilst suffering this grief, and hampered by my maladjusted way of dealing with it, was virtually impossible. At that time, even though not so long ago, it was much harder to access counselling or similar support and I didn't even know such help even existed. Following this I had several more close bereavements within quick succession, I became homeless and in 1992 had a major psychotic relapse.

# Chapter 10: Amphetamine Induced Psychosis

By the summer of 1992, I simply had my finger on the self destruct button and had turned into some kind of amphetamine gannet. I was a hardcore user on the frontline of the scene and in the greatest danger of becoming a casualty.

It is rather difficult for me to disclose the following events relating to my drug use at that time. There is a moderate degree of apprehension for me about reliving my experiences as I speak them to my co-author, as the memories are of pain but also I have an additional and greater fear that my reasons for disclosing certain details of this dark period will be misinterpreted. In our society there are people who are so misguided that they would speak of practices, such as I am about to tell of, in a manner that could fairly be considered bragging. I am not such a person and now wish to make it clear that I am only referring to any sordid details of drug use in order to paint an accurate picture of how negative in the extreme the whole affair was for me. My hope is that the reader will conclude that the whole business is a loser's game, but then this is neither under my control nor my responsibility and I leave that with you.

Masking my problems with frequent and large doses of amphetamine left me feeling, as I can best describe, feeling externally high but internally traumatised. Hurt had turned to pain, with leaving my wife and not seeing my son making me feel as though my heart and soul had been ripped out of me. Amphetamines are not an appropriate remedy for this affliction. Days would pass without me sleeping, often whist in the company of people who were more psychologically disturbed than myself, or who were morally dubious and in my vulnerable state I was susceptible to being influenced by any of my associates. I would frequently experience extremes of mood, both high and low, within a short space of time and unfortunately my disturbances were not even limited to my emotions as my thoughts were affected too. Soon my thinking was so disordered that I was compulsorily admitted to hospital with amphetamine psychosis.

Prior to admission, I had been injecting copious quantities of a variety of different forms of amphetamines and excessive dosing, to varying degrees, was a regular occurrence. There were no all night parties any more and I had drifted so far into the hardcore scene that I had left the world of using the drug for genuine socialising purposes well behind. Once upon a time I had been around a Northern Soul scene upon which occasionally one might use amphetamines to enhance the night. Later I had discovered an all night party scene with the socialising fuelled by the amphetamines, this drug being the lifeblood of the party, and now I was injecting amphetamines into my blood without a party-goer in sight. For company I had only a few haggard skeletons, mostly male, that vaguely resembled people that used to be party goers not so long ago. I had travelled, at speed (pardon the pun), from a life of fun and laughter into the eye of the storm. This representing my progression as an amphetamine user; I was at a more advanced stage in my journey. What was further down the road? Where was the final destination going to be?

The psychological addiction of amphetamines can be overwhelming enough alone but many users additionally fall victim to being psychologically addicted to the ritual of injecting and the association of the pain of the needle with what comes soon thereafter. If there is a high enough dose of actual amphetamines in the powder, or other medium, purchased the following experience would consist of an overpowering adrenaline rush, inescapable to mind, body and soul that is physically warming and lifts the mood to unnatural highs that nature never intended. It becomes very apparent to anyone who flies so high that later, in the absence of the drug that the unbelievable excruciating lows are also found inescapable by the mind, body and soul (a point that one may feel foolish and regretful about overlooking).

The hardcore members of this elite fraternity, as some of them would see it, who have survived the journey to the point at which they are currently at, tend to have their own value system which is an important part of the scene in which they are involved in and plays an important part in preventing many of them escaping it. They often see themselves as great wise men and/or cool and the more amphetamines they use the higher their status; with such folk often being hero worshipped by naive, less experienced amphetamine users. In short many of the things they do and encourage others to do in order to increase social standing within this scene, actually have a powerful reverse effect outside the scene. The mark of an experienced, hardcore amphetamine user is one that attracts stigmatisation from non-drug users. To compound the effect, the way such amphetamine users encourage each other to use more increases the amount of mental health problems amongst them, which as obviously carries its own stigma and yet people within this sub-section of the drug scene can even obtain higher status amongst their peers for having such issues. Very simply during this period I could not help but be influenced by the values of people that were causing me to bring two serious quality of life reducing forms of stigma upon myself.

An interesting collection of philosophies, ideas and notions about how to live ones life, not to mention political ideologies, could be found amongst these extreme amphetamine users. One of the first rules were that if you weren't injecting then you were a nobody, not really one of their number, you weren't as clever as them and your opinions didn't count. Apparently injecting was cleaner than any other route of admission and this was an obvious fact that any fool should know. Perhaps there was nothing dirty about the fact that all this was going on in the middle of an HIV and hepatitis epidemic? Amongst the general population, if an individual experienced delusions of grandeur they would be in danger of finding themselves studying the interior decor of a psychiatric ward, however, on this scene they were more likely to be hero worshipped. Someone who had failed to sleep for several days, due to substantial dosages and whom was touching on psychosis would often be seen as someone experiencing revelation with great wisdoms to impart upon the world or at least the chosen ones (other "'phet' 'eds'") that were ready to sit there and listen. The people of this scene would often see themselves as being extremely creative and this could lead to great works of art that were difficult to appreciate by non-amphetamine users, but then what would that matter because non-amphetamine users didn't know what they were about. Actually the actual creators of theses works of art didn't quite appreciate them the same themselves once the amphetamines had wore off. The same creative drive could also lead other diverse activities ranging from dismantling household appliances with great ideas about how useful this would be, to decorating projects.

Stories about things happening to motor bikes during their owner's prolonged amphetamine using phases were commonplace on the drugs scene and such gifted mechanics seemed to be in no short supply. Amongst such works of art that I remember was a car that was hand painted with a mixture of different coloured paint, found on a tip, that wasn't different colours after it had all been mixed together and this delicate brushwork was conducted under the illumination of a street lamp.

The artist neither owned the car nor gave his permission for its enhancement. Oh dear.

My attempts to keep the lid on my own psychosis ended with my lid being blown off as if used for some forlorn attempt to plug an active volcano. Visiting the local shop had become a horrific ordeal and it would be impossible to decipher in retrospect which aspects of my experiences there were simply paranoia and which were very real, resultant from the stigma brought on by the locals knowledge of my drug use and by their reactions to my unusual and conspicuous behaviour. It was simply the way of things that each aspect of this experience fuelled the others as is the case for any poor unfortunate whose mental health is spiralling downwards through drug use. My readmission to hospital, that was only non inevitable in the sense that I could have died instead, was caused by a culmination of painful experiences and my series of disastrous decisions in response which had a domino-like effect.

# Chapter 11: Early to bed early to rise

Suddenly I found myself in a new environment altogether. As there was no room at Rotherham District General, I was admitted to Doncaster Royal Infirmary. No longer was I shoulder to shoulder with hardcore amphetamine users indoctrinating me but on an unfamiliar psychiatric ward. I had never stayed at this hospital before, and my new companions were probably talking a whole heap more sense than those whose company I had just been evacuated from.

Initially I was very anxious about not knowing the rules in this strange place, upsetting the staff and being the victim of another Largactil squad and re-living a piece of history I would rather forget. I had been on a tremendous journey of recovery, covering ground that I never thought possible and then as a direct result of my own actions, I had regressed straight back to square one or worse. This was my opportunity to wallow in my own tremendous sense of failure. The staff of Rotherham that had me transferred to Doncaster told me I was going there because it was in the same health trust. Well trust wasn't a word in my vocabulary right then and it was an unfamiliar place that concealed hidden dangers. My fears were largely unfounded. In the initial phase of my stay meals were brought to my room and I was pretty much waited on. Ok it still wasn't the Ritz but the staff members were immeasurably more hospitable than I had anticipated.

It is possible that the reason for the great improvement in my treatment since my first stay as a psychiatric inpatient was at least in part because upon this second stay I was older. My co-author tells me he had a similar experience as he had a terrible time as an inpatient in the Eighties when he was young, but had a second stay many years later during which his treatment was akin to that of a guest at a five-star hotel. After a brief comparing of notes on the issue we both concluded that, although conditions seem to have improved since the Eighties, much of our better treatment was probably as a result of our more advanced years, meaning that we were more able to communicate with the nursing staff, thus making us easier to look after and older people are generally treated with more respect in society anyway.

Being initially transferred from Rotherham fuelled my paranoia somewhat at the outset as I was suspicious that it was not because the ward was full but just because they didn't want me there. The fact that my stay at Doncaster represented a significant improvement over my earlier one at Rotherham acted as more than adequate compensation for this. When I was eventually due to leave, staff there commented on the fact that I had been brought there with a staff escort and yet had been gentle as a pussycat. I cannot praise the nursing staff there enough and thanks to their good care I only needed to be there a few weeks in total.

My sister Cheryl came to a doctor's appointment and encouraged me to tell of my drug use, of which I had initially been concealing and this helped the doctors choose my successful course of treatment. Unfortunately my access battle for my son depended heavily on me being able to produce favourable psychiatric reports and this episode of illness did my case tremendous damage. At least a plus was that my mother, who was tremendously disapproving of drugs, forgave me upon my recovery from this episode. Ultimately I soon came out of hospital with a much better mental state; however, there had been significant consequences for this period of drug use and resultant illness.

## Chapter 12: Second amphetamine induced episode

There I was discharged after a very successful intervention, I had more experience of life and there seemed no reason why life could not be good from now on. However, the damage to my case for access to my son remained and there was another patch of my history that added to the burden of stigma that I had to carry. A history of being a psychotic amphetamine user carries a weighty stigma, the kind which makes some supposedly caring individuals and the authorities want to deny you contact with your children. The rights and wrongs of the related issues are very complex but, put simply, this stigma had a devastating impact upon me and acted as an impenetrable barrier to my recovery: A recovery that fate would otherwise have been offering to me on a plate.

I went back to work down London far too early to cope with the strain and upon my return the vultures were waiting for me, old amphetamine associates/wide-boys and with my morale at rock bottom they lured me straight back into the scene. They were not interested in the fact that I had lost a brother, access to my son, the despair I was going through and the despair I had previously been through due to amphetamines; all they were interested in was re-recruiting an ex-user back to the scene and in some cases regaining a customer. The good work of the Doncaster staff was wiped out in an instant.

## Stigma: Worse than Psychosis

By August bank holiday 1993 I had a major relapse. Whilst both intoxicated by amphetamines actually in my system at the time and starting with psychosis, I was involved in a fracas with someone who had harmed a female member of my family. I instantly knew I had gone too far and soon found myself on the run from the police. For a while I laid low in Bristol, but upon my return to Rotherham had plain clothes police knocking at my door who immediately arrested me. Whilst in the cells I was painfully delusional, believing that my son was in extreme danger and I guess I was being a rather difficult guest; it's a good job for them that the cell doors were so strong.

After several hours in the cells someone came to see me and in the midst of the chaotic delusional tangents that my mind was wandering off into, I had a lucid moment in which I realised this woman had come to assess my mental state. This could hardly be considered a psychiatric evaluation as she only peered through the cell door. At this time no one in their right mind would have willingly entered this cell which contained someone who was clearly not. The interior of the cell was designed to resist vandalism and I rather fancy I was giving them their toughest challenge yet; all this did nothing to aid my assessment and my case to see my son.

I remember how stressed my mother looked in the magistrate's court but still thinking that at least I would soon be going home with her. Imagine how I felt when told I was being placed on remand.

The vehicle taking me to my new temporary place of residence resembled an armoured truck and I hadn't a clue where we were going but remember there were many twists and turns after leaving the motorway.

After quite a journey I found myself in a secluded cell, on a prison hospital wing, with staff rushing in to inject me. I was successful in my attempt to resist them and they left with the doors closing firmly behind them while I went through amphetamine withdrawals for the next few days. The dehydration sweats and inability to sleep were more than I could possibly describe or do justice to in this book. Whilst still experiencing this, but after a few days, I saw the latch on the cell door open and I was passed water and had a conversation with the senior prison officer during which I agreed to be medicated but in a far more civilised way. I knew that I was very ill and was ready to take the medication but wondered why they hadn't tried talking to me in the first place. This was one experience that has led me to believe that the importance of communication cannot be underestimated in these kinds of circumstances.

Once on medication, I had a formal psychiatric assessment from a psychiatrist from Rotherham and I expect that this was for the purposes of the impending court case. It felt like a bit of a relief to see someone from Rotherham in my still semi-psychotic state, even though I had had very little prior contact with him. Unexpectedly on the day of my court case rather than having to appear in court, I was transferred to a low secure unit. This journey was very different with the prison staff being far more relaxed and making pleasant conversation throughout the journey. The low security unit happened to be in Rotherham where one of the first things I did was to ask to be screened for HIV and Hepatitis; thankfully I was clear. This particular secure unit had such a bad stigma attached to it that even my co-author tells me, here and now, that he is shocked to discover that it was only a low security unit. He says the way folk used to rave on about it was as though Hannibal Lecter was not just a fictional character and was staying there, the rest of the patients would consider him tame and if one of them should get out, there would be few survivors. It wasn't quite like that!

Whilst staying there I encountered some of the staff from the old Largactil squad and was initially concerned that history would be repeated. Thankfully this was not the case, as the regular medication I was prescribed was working better than before and these people had got to know me more which improved communication. Although I didn't know any of the other patients at first, I soon became friendly with a few who I would play pool with and generally pass the time with. Whilst staying here I helped disarm someone who held a nurse hostage with a knife but the rest of the time was less eventful. Still weighing heavily on my mind was the whole business of how my court case would go and how this would impact on access to my son. Meanwhile other patients were appearing in court and not coming back, being detained for long periods under the Mental Health Act. This was a bad omen as a similar fate would damage my chances of ever being able to see my son.

The charge laid against me had been one of assault but was dropped by my accuser before the case was due to be heard, which was good news, but my solicitor came to see me to give me a warning. He told me that I had a bad reputation which could be problematic should I run into further trouble in the future and made his point very clear; I listened to him and took this on board. It had been the only time I had ever spent on a secure unit and following this I had no further clashes with the law or stays on psychiatric wards. This represented a significant turning point for me. At this point I would like to dispel the myth that if someone on a serious charge declares they have a mental illness or it is discovered that they have one that they somehow get an easy ride and escape justice. This is definitely not the case. Someone with a mental illness can easily find themselves detained for longer. A mentally healthy prisoner normally knows their release date whereas a patient on a secure unit does not and when a person is released from a secure unit the reputation they carry and stigma they have to bear is usually weightier than that of a mentally healthy ex-convict.

Upon my release from the secure unit, I went to stay with my elder sister and this was a time to reflect on my circumstances. I realised I had to act immediately and radically in order to turn my life around. It was so obvious that the worst evil that had been in my life and greatest threat to my future was amphetamine sulphate; a strong decision had to be made. From this time onwards I was never again to insult my body or mind with that vile substance. It was a very lonely journey as the greatest withdrawals I had to endure were caused by having to detox myself from the amphetamine using sub-culture and leave behind the parties and all night conversations. This was a point at which I had to socially start again, as my friends and associates had virtually all been drug users.

My father encouraged me to attend psychiatric outpatient appointments, getting all the help the system was ready to give me and all the rest of my family were extremely supportive during this period. Samantha, my youngest sister, also attended my outpatient appointments and encouraged me to get a key-worker to help me function out in the community. Although I felt stigmatised and thought nobody would want to know me, within a few months I found myself in a relationship with a woman I had known previously. With the aid of my family, my partner and my key-worker I made good progress on my journey of recovery. Instead of squandering money on drugs I spent it on sensible and constructive things even spending a little on my partner, saving up for the odd holiday. At this time I was taking all the help I could get for the first time ever, rather than trying to be the tough guy and deal with everything myself and as a result the momentum of my recovery was growing. At the same time as I was making this recovery, the court battle for access to my son was underway. Unfortunately it was not going well but thankfully, with the help of all around me, this was not enough to push me into a relapse.

All the court hearings had been delayed due to me having been ill previously but now the whole business was fully underway. The court welfare office was very helpful and supportive during this period. After the court hearings were over, this court welfare officer explained to me how I would not be allowed to see my son because of my mental health problems. Although this was a personal disaster to me, something constructive did come from it, as this man inspired me to maximise my recovery and after hearing about my experiences and that fact that I was considering writing a book pointed out that I was able to laugh at it all looking back. I was definitely in a more positive frame of mind and in fact I remember my sister Samantha saying that I had to think positive and now it has become a feeling and not just a word.

My life had changed such that bills actually got paid and my increase in ability to be organised changed so many aspects of my life. A great deal of support was given to me here by my key-worker, it took several years of their patience but their labours paid off. The greatest motivational force to encourage me to recover was the thought that the more well I was the better chance I would have of one day seeing my son and I knew that if I became ill rumours could travel around town and reach even him making him wary of ever meeting me. Through the next few years my family experienced more than its fair share of trauma but we all stuck together to battle on through the best we could and at least, as a consolation, it gave me chance to give something back in terms of support.

The cumulative support of all around me had done its job and soon I could not imagine ever slipping back into the drug scene, the pain lay behind me and a new adventure ahead. I started to live a lifestyle that incorporated many of the more conventional pleasures that people enjoy and took advantage of many opportunities that society has to offer to its more functional members. Passing my driving test was one simple event that opened up new opportunities to improve my quality of life.

## Chapter 13: Introducing Beyond The Cuckoo's Nest, by Martin

Just after the millennium Jason had a change of key-worker. At first he was sceptical as the previous one had been great but the new one would also turn out to be so too. She said he had made a great degree of recovery, had plenty to talk about and she made him aware of a voluntary mental health educational organisation called "Beyond the Cuckoo's Nest". This organisation's purpose was to address and challenge ignorance, negative stereotypes and stigma surrounding mental health issues and the method employed was to hold workshops in the community. The format of these workshops was such that approximately half of the time was allocated to mental health service-users giving their own personal testimonies of their experiences. It was intended that if people out in the community met real life people who had experienced mental illness they would become more enlightened and more empathic about such phenomena. Well this organisation was in need of recruiting more mental health service-users as speakers and talking is something Jason does very readily. He also has the ability to recall with humour events that would so obviously have been very traumatic at the time, making any speech a little entertaining, more easy listening and lighter than the horror story that it could be.

Around about the mid-nineties a small group of Mental Health Services staff, working in

Rotherham, were awarded funding for a trip to Canada to see how the Canadian services worked. Whilst there they came across an organisation called "Beyond The Cuckoo's Nest" that conducted educational workshops about mental health issues and delivered their service to massive audiences. The Rotherham Mental Health Services staff was so impressed they decided to import the idea to Britain. After gaining permission from the Canadians to use the same project name Beyond The Cuckoo's Nest Rotherham was set up. It was necessary to make a few adaptations to better tailor it to the South Yorkshire catchment area it was to serve, with targeting smaller audiences and making it more personal possibly being the main differences. It soon caught on and other Beyond The Cuckoo's Nests were formed in other areas of the country with a particularly large one in Birmingham at one point. These organisations ran for a while but at the date of writing this book only the Rotherham Beyond The Cuckoo's Nest is still running.

Firstly Jason went along to a workshop as an observer to get a flavour of how they worked and determine whether it was for him. Straight away it appealed as here was an opportunity to speak of his experiences to a mostly interested audience and do some good for a cause relevant to him at the same time. Jason enjoys recounting the odd yarn anyway and here was a golden opportunity. Jason immediately made the decision to join there and then in autumn 2002 and has done an awful lot of talking since. To Jason, as with many others involved with Beyond The Cuckoo's Nest, it represented empowerment in that it offered an opportunity to use painful experiences from the past that were self esteem lowering and make constructive use of them, thus raising self esteem and there was also the opportunity to develop skills at doing this.

Jason has delivered his talks to many people over the last few years and in addition to appreciation shown at the time has had numerous instances of very positive feedback. For example Jason would often be involved in workshops delivered to audiences of 6th form students and one time he was approached by a student psychiatric nurse who told him that he had been inspired to choose this career path after hearing him speak when he was in the 6th form: This young man is now a qualified psychiatric nurse.

A couple of teacher friends of Jason's invited him to speak about his experiences at their schools where he went and gave his testimony representing his organisation. Beyond The Cuckoo's Nest offered Jason a wealth of new positive experiences which helped combat the damage done by the stigma that had burdened him through so much of his life as they raised his self esteem. This organisation filled Jason with confidence and was a major contributor to his inspiration to write his first book; a project which he worked on concurrently. In that book he described the massive positive impact it had on his life.

## Stigma: Worse than Psychosis

It was during his time working with Beyond The Cuckoo's Nest and whilst still working on his first book that I met Jason. That is to say the first time I was aware of meeting him as we could easily have met years previously in the circles we moved in whilst too smashed to have the faintest clue who we had been introduced to or just spoke to. He seemed to be enjoying his life after drug abuse, life after hospital and life after stigma or at least the worst ravages of it. There will always be people who remember him for his mental illness but their memories will be growing more distant and Jason had largely beaten the worst of the damaging effects of the stigma by gaining control over his self image. His personal battle seemed to have largely been won as he was all smiles and grins with many positive things to say and has remained this way for most of the time I have known him.

He was always keen to support other mental health service users wherever he met them and offer his hard learned wisdoms to anyone who might benefit. One particular conversation I had with him sticks in my mind as it really helped me find the way forward when I was wrestling with a rather difficult conundrum and he surprised me with his insight. Often the experiences a psychosis suffer has are very similar to many of the experiences of other such sufferers but the individuals concerned are frequently too terrified to speak of them. Well it seems that Jason has overcome such fear. He has had quite an extreme taste of psychosis and can relate well to most other suffers. When I first met him, upon joining Beyond

The Cuckoo's Nest myself, I learned much about his past straight away through his willingness to speak frankly. Soon I heard him speaking with the same frankness to other service users involved in the project, sometimes in the form of exchanging notes so to speak and sometimes giving advice. It is of no surprise to me that he now finds himself in a supporting role working with early psychosis sufferers whom have often become ill at a similar age to himself and whom have sometimes had a similar lifestyle.

## Chapter 14: Early Intervention in Psychosis

After struggling to see my son for fourteen years and being in recovery for over a decade, by 2004, we became reunited around his sixteenth birthday with help from his grandparents. This was a significant morale boost and a well needed one as it coincided with the break-up of yet another relationship. I had been determined for many years that should I get to see him again, he would see me in a mentally healthy state which would help counter the effects of any negative rumours he might have heard about me.

Approximately six months later, by the end of the same year, I passed the interview for a new job but received a letter telling me not to bother going for my medical health check. Due to the employers knowing something about my mental health in advance they decided that I was not suitable for the job. A few months later, at a Beyond The Cuckoo's Nest meeting, I was informed that the local mental health service were willing to recruit people who had been service-users to become "Support Time and Recovery workers (STAR workers)". By November 2005 I had been through the interview process and secured a post as a STAR worker with the "Rotherham Early Intervention in Psychosis Team"; also simply known as the "Early Intervention Team" (EIT). As fate would have it the work place where I was refused a job because of my mental health history closed down around this time and so things had worked out for the better. I acquired a mortgage which was one of my goals at this time and was surprised when the home insurance went up from the original quote after I disclosed that I had previous mental health issues.

The Rotherham EIT is a family oriented team which aims to provide non-stigmatised care and support to those aged between 14 and 35 years old who are experiencing first episode psychosis. Importantly it attempts to reduce the duration of untreated illness and place the focus on recovery and independence. I really wished there had been something like this around for me when I was younger, as I felt proud to be on board and immediately saw the potential for great job satisfaction. It was interesting working in a multi-disciplinary team as I met many people with different knowledge and skills and later on even found myself in the company of my co-author again as he was based there for his research project for his Masters degree. It was then that we decided to write this book together.

In April 2006 I won the chairman's award for the Rotherham, Doncaster and South Humber health authority on the 10th Anniversary of the creation of this award for special inspiration as regards my recovery and my work with the EIT was a large influence towards this happening. Prior to this I had been apprehensive about how I would fit into the team and was very self-conscious about the fact that I had been a severe psychosis sufferer and I was now involved with a myriad of professionals that were mostly just used to relating to psychosis suffers as patients. Would they respect or listen to me? Well thankfully I received a wealth of positive feedback including praise about sharing my insider views of psychosis and being able to relate to clients that were otherwise difficult because of my insights.

Whilst working in this post I have had to study at Doncaster College to gain my Certificate in Mental Health Level Three and undertake a couple of shorter courses and I would like to thank my friends and colleagues who supported me through this period. It had been a long time since I had studied and at the beginning I had my anxieties about this. These qualifications were necessary to equip me with the skills needed to be effective in this post. Soon I was interacting with the whole team in the process whereby everyone gave their specialised input into planning and executing care interventions for clients and their families. Soon I knew I had found my spiritual home.

In May 2007, at the last match of the season at my hometown Rotherham United Football Club I was honoured guest to launch my autobiography Sex, Drugs and Northern Soul. My publisher, and friend, Jason Pegler, CEO of Chipmunka Publishing, supported me at my launch, which received positive local media coverage. I can remember the days when people would cross on the other side of the road to avoid me due to my mental health problems, so it shows you how far we have come in terms of discrimination; however, there is still room for improvement. My colleagues at work and the trust I am employed by fully support anti-stigma initiatives, and part of my role is to help empower people to overcome their anxieties about stigma.

I was to find that my role also involved promoting social inclusion and recovery, including taking people out into the community to engage in various activities from day to day from things like shopping to recreational pursuits like playing snooker. Helping clients with claiming benefits, reassuring them, giving them a chance to discuss their issues, helping them access services and helping them with all aspects of their lives that their illness made difficult would all turn out to be part of my role. Some similar help had been given to me as a young man but this went the extra mile and the input was at the stage of illness at which it would have the most benefit. I thought this was great, I am still working in this post at the time of writing this book and can bear testimony to the importance of Early Intervention in psychosis. In my personal experience I have seen a much greater tendency for favourable outcomes the earlier a first episode psychosis sufferer is referred to the team. About eighteen months ago I had my duties expanded, being made a drug link worker, which allows me to make further use of my personal experiences and of course this pleases me no end.

## Summary: by Jason

Being able to talk about what happened to me in the past, gave me more of a feeling of control over my life than I ever had. A lot of times when you're not well, your mental health problems are only ever described or put into words by the people around you, the psychiatrists, social workers, nurses or your family. The psychiatrist diagnoses what's wrong with you, gives you a label and decides what medication you're going to get. The nurses or social workers tell you what you need to do to change, because a lot of the time in their eyes it's you that needs to change not the world around you. Then your family have their views on why they think you became unwell, why you behaved in this or that way. It doesn't matter how many times you're assessed or counselled, no-one can really know what's going on inside your head and no one can really walk in your shoes. They can't know what experiences you've had in life and how they've affected you, the knocks, and the setbacks. Everyone is different and everyone reacts in their own way to the things that life can throw at you.

Writing this book gave me the chance to talk about my life and my mental health problems in my own words. You could say it gave me a sense of having some control over my history; setting the record straight in some ways. Seeing my life written out across the pages chronologically also helped me to make sense of how things have worked out. I can see all the good things I've done over the years and I'm proud of them and regret nothing, but I can also see the points where I took the wrong path, made a wrong decision, and how these contributed to the difficulties I've experienced. In a way it's like coming to terms with things and that's positive because then you can start moving on, like I have done. You have more a feeling of being able to control your own destiny. I now feel I have broken free of the chains of stigma that have held me back so much in my life. They say you can't beat the illness but then again the illness has never beaten me. There's life after drug abuse and hospital and I'm here to say that! What stigma?

Lightning Source UK Ltd.
Milton Keynes UK
UKOW051339300512

193635UK00001B/23/P